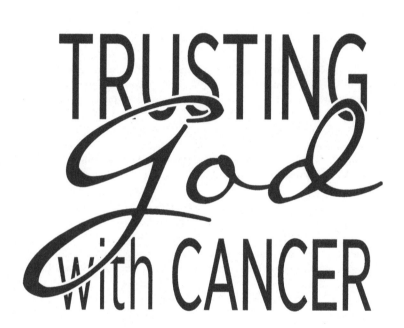

ROB RABAN

Trusting God with Cancer

Copyright © 2018 by Rob Raban

Published in the United States by Rob Raban LLC.

Edited by Lisa Guest

Formatting by Christian Editing Services (www.christianeditingservices.com)

Unless otherwise indicated, Scripture quotations are taken from *The Holy Bible, New International Version®*, **NIV® Copyright © 1973, 1978, 1984, 2011 by Biblica, Inc.® Used by permission. All rights reserved worldwide.**

Scripture quotations marked ESV are from *The English Standard Version*. © 2001 by Crossway Bibles, a division of Good News Publishers. Used by permission.

Scripture quotations marked NLT are from *Holy Bible, New Living Translation*. © 1996, 2004, 2007, 2013. Used by permission of Tyndale House Publishers, Inc., Carol Stream, Ill. 60188. All rights reserved.

Scripture quotations marked NKJV are from *The New King James Version*. © 1982 by Thomas Nelson, Inc. Used by permission. All rights reserved.

LIBRARY OF CONGRESS CATALOGUING-IN-PUBLICATION DATA

Raban, Rob.

Trusting God with Cancer / Rob Raban

ISBN 9780692920787

For my beloved wife, Barbi,

and sons Austin, Spencer, and Colby,

whose love inspired me to fight for my life

and to trust God with everything.

CONTENTS

FOREWORD

My hope for this book is to help you beat cancer and, in the process, know God more fully and trust Him to carry your burden.

I know that a diagnosis of cancer can be frightening. *Extremely frightening.* Diagnosed with Stage 4 T-cell lymphoma when I was thirty-nine and forced to face the possible loss of my loving wife and three young sons, I know a lot about being frightened! After all, every one of us knows people who haven't survived cancer; I have lost several dear friends to this cruel disease. But I also know that there's greater hope for a cure than ever before. More and more people are beating cancer each and every day.

As a cancer survivor, I feel called by God to pass along the kind of encouragement I received, the wisdom I gained, and the strategies I learned. I want to help you face cancer and beat it. And while cancer is scary and pregnant with all sorts of emotions and fears, I can also tell you that I am better off for the experience. Too many blessings have come out of the journey. So, while it is natural to fear the worst, if you're open to it, you will also find some amazing blessings along the way, one of which just may be a personal encounter with God Almighty.

Regardless of your faith, regardless of your beliefs, regardless of your convictions, regardless of your ethnicity, regardless of any other distinctions by which one can categorize us human beings, there is one undeniable truth: *cancer* can strike anyone.

If you are facing cancer or any other life-threatening disease, there is also a corresponding truth you absolutely need to know: ***nothing is bigger than God.***

Chapter 1

Misdiagnosing a Sneeze

I'D JUST ARRIVED HOME FROM A BUSINESS TRIP AND NEEDED to repack quickly so I could catch the shuttle boat to Catalina Island. It was mid-October, 2001, and the weather was perfect. I was looking forward to being the best man at a close friend's wedding. After a quick kiss "hello" to my wife, Barbi, I raced upstairs to my bedroom and began packing.

I have two rows of hangers on my side of the closet, and my shirts are on the upper bar. As I reached up to grab a shirt, I sneezed. *Oww!! That hurt!* Since I was in a hurry, I didn't process the degree of the pain. It just registered that somewhere under my right arm, it hurt—and I was late. With a quick "goodbye" kiss for Barbi and the boys, I was off, racing to Long Beach and the boat for Catalina and the wedding.

During the course of the weekend, the pain in my ribs more or less subsided, but there was always a dull, nagging feeling. Soon after I got home from Catalina, I made an appointment to see my primary care doctor. I had HMO insurance and, up to that point, had been satisfied with it. I liked my doctor, and I could generally see him whenever I wanted to see him. In the examining room, Dr. Barnes (not his real name) felt around under my arm, poked and prodded a bit, and discovered that I had indeed cracked a rib. *My sneeze had cracked my rib?*

"This can't be common," I said to the doctor. He informed me that it happens more often than one would think.

Unfortunately, there's not a lot anyone can do for cracked ribs, so his prescription was simple: "Take it easy and take Tylenol for pain when needed."

Over the next few weeks as the pain diminished, I went about my life. I was happily married, and Barbi and I had just recently celebrated our twelfth wedding anniversary. We have three sons, and at the time of my cracked rib, my oldest son Austin was nine, Spencer was seven, and Colby was five.

I love my boys and I love playing sports, so to have three boys to come home to and wrestle around and play sports with is just about the most amazing thing a dad could ever ask for. And at this point in their lives, Dad was still king. I was still admired and, in their eyes, still a great athlete. Teenage pessimism—when Dad loses some of his luster— was a few years away, so while I was still wanted, I took this opportunity to be as much involved as possible in their various sports activities.

Little League season was coming up soon, and the boys wanted to break out their mitts and start warming up for baseball season. Unfortunately, with my sore rib, I found it more than a little painful to throw the ball and play catch.

However, there was a community pool in our housing tract, so the boys and I would regularly hit the pool and relax in the warmth of the Jacuzzi. These visits to the Jacuzzi were a nice, restful substitute for our regular playtime. But something more than my sore rib was bothering me....

What Is Going On?

I was tired.

Now, as a husband, the father of three young boys, an active member at church, and vice president of our small family business, I was always busy. I figured that my fatigue was the natural result of managing all those responsibilities and not getting much exercise since the day I broke my rib. So I vowed to make time to work out and see if I could regain some stamina.

As the days rolled on, I began to sense that something was going on under my right arm besides a cracked rib. I remember telling Barbi it felt "spongy" under my arm. She urged me to see the doctor again, report my latest symptoms, and get some tests run. I made another appointment and shared with Dr. Barnes that I was dealing with intermittent pain under my arm, that it felt "spongy," and that Barbi wanted me to get it checked out. After feeling around under my arm for a few moments, Dr. Barnes said a bit condescendingly "to tell your wife that you have a blocked sweat duct and to change deodorants." No other tests were ordered. I went home and told Barbi my diagnosis. "That's weird," I remember her saying. And we both just kind of let it go.

The holidays came and went—busy, busy, busy—and tryouts for spring baseball were underway. I was looking forward to coaching my son Colby's T-ball team just as I had coached T-ball for his two older brothers. But the thought of adding coaching responsibilities to my already busy life wasn't appealing. I was tired. *I* was tired? Something was definitely wrong. I love coaching, but just thinking about a season full of practices and games was draining. And that strange feeling, that intermittent pain underneath my arm, was not getting better. So I made another trip to the doctor's office.

"Broken ribs take a while to heal," Dr. Barnes reiterated.

"But what about the pain under my arm?" I asked. "I'm not even using deodorant, so that can't be causing any issues. And sometimes the pain goes across my chest. Isn't it unusual for these symptoms to last this long?"

"Not really," he said. Again, I went home with nothing new to report to my wife.

Another symptom that had been going on—a symptom the doctor failed to ask me about and I failed to volunteer— was night sweats. I didn't think anything of them. I would get them from time to time, and I just thought it was because of our down comforter that my wife prefers. It can be a bit hot for me.

It wasn't long, however, before the night sweats became more frequent and were becoming more intense. I was literally soaking through two T-shirts per night and had to lie on a towel so the sheets wouldn't get soaked. I explained away this occurrence, letting myself think the sweating was due to recent heat spells and a house that wasn't air conditioned.

"Something's wrong," Barbi said. "We need to demand some tests. Aren't there some x-rays or something they can do to find out what's going on inside?"

I was not in the mood for another appointment with my doctor. I had already seen him three times for ostensibly the same thing, and I did not want to waste time visiting him again.

A Surprising Comment

When I went to work the next day, I got a call from a sales rep who wanted to come by, say hello, and discuss a little business for a manufacturer he was representing. "No problem, Tom," I said. "Come on by."

When Tom arrived, the first thing he said to me was "Are you feeling OK? You look tired."

Now, I hadn't seen Tom in quite a while, and the fact that he noticed immediately that I looked tired struck me. "You know, Tom, I feel tired," I said.

Intuition—that funny feeling, the odd thought, the comment that won't go away, the proverbial gut feeling that certain business leaders swear by before they sign off on a deal—works in strange ways, but I think it's one of the ways God communicates with us to help us along. With Tom's comment, a variety of intuitions, strange feelings, and odd thoughts came together and started calling to me. I shared Tom's comments and my feelings with Barbi.

"I told you, something *is* going on," she repeated. And something *was* going on. Even though I had been exercising more, I was still tired, and near-strangers who rarely saw me quickly recognized the fatigue in me. With Colby's baseball season getting underway and my once again being head coach, I needed to figure out what I was battling, or I wouldn't have the energy to coach. I had rationalized for months that it was normal for someone in my busy stage of life to feel tired. I had seen the doctor several times for the same thing and always heard the same diagnosis: "You're a busy dad with a cracked rib. It will get better with time." Well, it wasn't getting better with time. My body was trying to tell me something and I needed to become a better advocate for my health.

Full Swing

During the course of the same day that Tom commented on my fatigue, Barbi and her friend Jennifer happened to be watching *Terms of Endearment,* a tearjerker movie that deals with cancer and loss. "Jennifer!" Barbi said. "Something is very wrong with Rob. I just know it."

When I got home from work, Barbi called me into the family room. "Rob, you need to see Dr. Barnes tomorrow and demand some x-rays." I had no idea if Barbi thought I had cancer. She hadn't said that to me, but she knew something was wrong. With my fatigue and underarm pain not getting better, it was abundantly clear that I needed some tests.

"I'll do it," I said. I made the appointment, went into the Dr. Barnes's office, and firmly stated my case: "I'm tired. I'm not getting better. I need some x-rays and whatever tests are necessary to find out what's going on." Dr. Barnes agreed and sent me to radiology. Finally, I got some x-rays taken and was hopeful we'd find out what was going on. I would have to wait a few days for the results.

At home, things were getting into full swing for baseball season. Yes, I had taken on the coaching responsibilities for Colby's team despite the fatigue I felt. I didn't want to miss out on one of the great joys of being a father: I got to coach my son. Yet coaching your own child can be one of the hardest things in the world to do because—let's face it—sometimes our kids don't want to listen to us. But compliance was not at all an issue for five-year-old Colby, and Dad was still a hero. We began practicing with the team, playing catch, hitting off the batting tee, and learning the game. I also realized that even though Colby writes with his right hand, he's a lefty on the baseball field. That means, among other things, that when he stands at the plate to hit, he's one step closer to first base.

Austin and Spence were also playing baseball, Austin in Minor B and Spencer in Minor C. The season was just getting started when I got a call from the doctor's office. My test results were in. "We've found something," Dr. Barnes said.

Chapter 2

"Your Cancer Is Doubling on the Hour"

"YOUR RIGHT SEVENTH RIB LOOKS CHEWED UP," DR. BARNES said after examining my x-rays.

"Chewed up? I repeated. "What does that mean?"

"I'm sending you to Hoag Hospital to run more tests and find out exactly what it does mean."

The fact that the doctor was referring me out for more tests was a strong indication that the actual diagnosis wasn't a broken rib or a blocked sweat gland!

Barbi and I drove to Hoag Hospital in Newport Beach for our morning appointment. We filled out forms, had copies of my driver's license and insurance card made, and then were shown to the radiology waiting room. Barbi and I joined hands and prayed for comfort and protection. A friendly young nurse named Virginia introduced herself and escorted me back to the room where the procedure would be performed.

A bone marrow or needle core biopsy is the removal of a small piece (about 2cm x 0.16 cm) of intact bone marrow. Blood cells are made in the bone marrow, and a biopsy is taken to either rule out or confirm various types of cancer, such as leukemia, Hodgkin's disease, and non-Hodgkin's lymphoma. I didn't know any of this at the time, however. I only knew I was getting more tests done to find out what was going on with me.

I was first taken to a small locker room where I undressed and put on a hospital gown. Then I was shown to a bed, given a mild sedative, wheeled into an operating room, and transferred to the operating table. One of the nurses opened the gown at my chest and wiped me down with an antiseptic. A surgically masked doctor explained that he would puncture first my skin and then my sternum to extract some bone marrow samples. He held in his hand what appeared to be an industrial-grade staple gun. I was told to raise my arms over my head in order to fully expose my chest. Though I was somewhat relaxed from the sedative I'd been given, it still was quite a vulnerable feeling to have all these doctors and nurses standing above me and not have my arms for protection. But then an amazing thing happened.

A Helping Hand

With my arms raised above and my chest laid bare, the doctor readied the cold, stainless steel staple gun, placed it against my sternum, and prepared to fire his first shot. I braced myself for pain and was about to squeeze my outstretched hands into a fist when, to my surprise, someone squeezed back!

BAM!! The doctor pulled the trigger, and the staple (actually a needle) penetrated my chest, went through my sternum and into my bone marrow— I winced in pain. But at that exact moment of contact, at that split second of pain, there—smiling above me—was my nurse Virginia, and her hands were squeezed in with mine. I don't remember the degree of pain I felt, but I do remember the degree of care I felt when the biopsy needle entered my chest and Virginia absorbed the first shot with me.

Thinking about this now, I am overcome with emotion and gratitude for Virginia's care. With three more staple shots to come, boy, did I need a hand to hold onto! I couldn't use my arms to protect myself, and the fear and my sense of vulnerability were suffocatingly real—and *that's* when she squeezed my hand. Virginia's care was every bit as important to me as the care the seasoned doctors, full of knowledge, experience, and degrees, provided me on the operating table. God used Virginia's hand to help me stare down a room full of steel and uncertainty… and feel secure. God was also delivering a crucial message to me at that moment: He made it clear to me that He would comfort me and protect me, that I would not fight this battle alone.

> *"As a mother comforts her child, so will*
> *I comfort you."*
>
> God's promise in Isaiah 66:13

In Sickness and in Health...

The most powerful armament God gave me here on this earth is my wife. I could not have faced this battle without Barbi. During the anxious moments, hours, and days that passed before we learned our test results, Barbi was resolute in following up with Dr. Barnes's office. When Dr. Barnes's office told Barbi the results weren't in, she called Hoag's radiology lab. Hoag said that the results had already been sent over to Dr. Barnes's office and to check back with them. Barbi called his office again saying that Hoag told her the results were already sent over to them and asked if they could please check again. The nurse said the doctor would be checking results and making call backs at 6:00 p.m. after patient visits. Six p.m. came and went. No call.

With our family and friends praying for us and wanting to know what was going on, Barbi called the doctor's office when it opened the following morning. Calmly saying that she hadn't heard from the doctor the evening before, she respectfully asked the office nurse to please double-check to see if our results were in, explaining again what Hoag radiology had told her the day before. Without even checking, the office nurse snapped, "We'll get to it when we get to it. What makes you think your husband's test results are more important than anyone else's?"

Barbi was in no mood for this!

"Do you mean to tell me that someone coming in with a common cold is as high a priority as someone waiting for the results of a potentially life-threatening disease?" Barbi asked incredulously.

"We treat all of our patients equally," said the nurse.

Barbi asked her if she could simply walk over to the inbox to confirm if our results were there. The nurse refused and hung up the phone.

A few moments later, the doctor called Barbi back, not with the test results or to apologize for misdiagnosing my condition for six months, but with an admonishment to stop harassing his nurses with questions about test results they didn't have. "I wasn't harassing your nurses, Doctor. I was simply asking them to do their job. I was promised a call from you last night and never received one. I also checked with radiology at Hoag, and they confirmed with a stamped time receipt that your office got the results *yesterday*. Are you saying these test results are not a priority and you refuse to simply walk over to your inbox to check?"

Dr. Barnes stated, "All my patients are important, and I will get to it when I get to it."

An hour later Barbi received another call from the flustered, yet still unapologetic doctor to say that the test results were in. "You can tell your husband that he has T-cell lymphoma. I'm referring you to an oncologist."

Barbi's frustration—from the six months of my going to see this doctor and his missing all the signs that I had something more serious than sore ribs, her frustration with the fact that *we* had to insist on getting further tests, and, after we got these tests done, her frustration with the doctor's failure to treat her husband's case with appropriate urgency and get back to us in a timely manner—came to a head.

"No, Dr. Barnes! *You* will be a professional, and *you* will tell Rob yourself!" Barbi said. "You also need to call and make the oncologist appointment for us—and make sure we get in this afternoon." There were no further protestations from the doctor.

I was at work in my office when I received Dr. Barnes's call. I had been anxiously waiting two days for the news. I had T-cell lymphoma, and he had made an appointment for me to see an oncologist, Dr. Collins (not her real name). He added, "I'd go to her if I had your diagnosis."

I was stunned. All I knew was that I had to hang up the phone, get out of my office, and get home as fast as I could. One thought grabbed my attention, and I couldn't shake it: "I don't want to die."

Once in the car—and ready to crack, I immediately called Barbi for support and blurted the news of my diagnosis. Barbi cut in: "I know, I know. I'm so sorry, Rob... That Dr. Barnes! I want to..."

"Barbi!" I interrupted. "Don't go there. I can't invest any emotion in him!"

Our conversation skipped a beat. I knew that Barbi needed to release her emotions, her fears, her anger, but so did I. I needed to tell Barbi how scared I was and that I needed her. But I couldn't explain that now. I was too upset. *This isn't about you!* I thought, not realizing at the time that in fact it was about both of us. If I check out and Barbi is left to raise three boys on her own, this cancer was definitely about both of us!

Finally, Barbi said, "OK, Rob. I'll meet you at the oncologist's office."

Our appointment with Dr. Collins was for three o'clock

that afternoon. I have absolutely no memory of how I got there, but what happened in the doctor's office is something I will never forget.

We were sitting in the examination room when the doctor came in—*we* being Barbi, me, and our longtime family friend Karen Koeller, whom Barbi had had the foresight to bring along.

Before becoming a stay-at-home mom, Karen worked as an oncology nurse. She had spent several years working in the pediatric oncology ward at UCLA's Ronald Reagan Hospital. We were unaware of what lay ahead, but Karen knew the terrain and the questions to ask. Her knowledge and perspective would be greatly needed and would prove very helpful.

"This Cancer Is Not Bigger Than God!"

A bespectacled Dr. Collins arrived with my patient file in hand. She politely introduced herself and then took a moment to review the paperwork. A petite woman with a quiet demeanor, she looked up after reading my file and haltingly began to tell me about my diagnosis.

"The tests show that you have T-cell lymphoma, non-Hodgkins. It is very aggressive. We need to start chemotherapy immediately."

"How aggressive?" I asked.

"Your cancer is doubling on the hour," she replied.

Someone in the room gasped.

I started to imagine cancer cells splitting and doubling,

splitting and doubling. *Dear Lord!* I quickly put the thought—
that image—out of my mind.

"Is it curable?" asked Barbi. "What is the survival rate?"

Dr. Collins hesitated before reciting some mortality
statistics that were anything but helpful or encouraging. I
noticed Barbi's left arm begin to tremble. She hesitatingly
asked Dr. Collins, "What... what do we tell our children?"

"Cancer is usually hardest on children of the same sex as
the cancer patient," she explained. The doctor then looked at
our file.

"You have three boys," she noted. "I also have three boys."
And with that simple statement, Dr. Collins began to cry.

Now I'm sure Dr. Collins was crying out of compassion
for me, for my family, and for these dire circumstances
we suddenly found ourselves in, but I had no place for
her sympathy. Barbi's trembling arm began to shake
uncontrollably as the weight of what we were facing became
unmistakably clear. *Was this it for me? Was it my time to go?
Was I going to die?...*

A tidal wave of emotions flooded in: an intense fear of
dying, an intense sadness over losing my boys, and then
came anger over what felt like my being written off as
good as dead—but it was my beloved wife's quivering arm
and my compassion for her that shot me to my feet with a
determination I could taste. I wasn't going to accept this! I
would fight for her! I would fight for us!

"Doctor," I sat upright and boldly asked, "is there a cure
rate to this?"

"Yes, there is a cure rate," she acknowledged.

"Well, I don't care if it's 1%, I'm going to be that 1%! This cancer is not bigger than God!" I exclaimed. "If it's my time to go, then it's my time to go, but God is not afraid of this cancer—and we're not going to run in fear of it!"

I asked everyone to stand up with me and join hands. So Barbi, Karen, and Dr. Collins stood with me, and I prayed, giving my disease over to God, acknowledging His sovereignty over my life and His power to cure me in an instant. And in that moment everything changed. No longer clammy, fearful, and flushed, I felt resolute. With 100% certainty, I knew that God could win this fight. I firmly believed that God *could* cure me.

Standing up and speaking boldly while leading others in prayer was definitely **not** my personality. But there was something about Barbi's quivering arm, her naked, vulnerable trembling. It was so *pure* and so pained. She couldn't hide or disguise her fear, and my heart broke. In sheer desperation I cried out to God. I didn't think about what I found myself doing. I didn't strategize about it. I didn't weigh my options, my sins, my faults, or any good things I've done to deserve God's help.

Like David, I just cried out to Him:

> *In my distress I called upon the Lord,*
> *And cried out to my God;*
> *He heard my voice from His temple,*
> *And my cry came before Him, even to His ears.*

> Psalm 18:6 NKJV

And God *did* help me. He used my cancer to get me off my butt and, when my life was on the line, proclaim my belief in Him. God allowed the painful reality of my wife's arm, shaking uncontrollably, to anchor for me the reality of what I was facing. God allowed me to be fully present in the most painful moment of my life so that my eyes could be fully opened. And in that moment *I fully believed in God!* I truly believed—not intellectually, not logically, I daresay not even in faith, but I believed with solid conviction and total certainty. Far from abandoning me during this horrible disease, God was showing me how real His power and presence are. God heard my cry for help and responded.

When your life is totally on the line, who will you reach out to?

> *"The LORD is my strength and my shield;*
> *my heart trusts in him, and he helps me."*
>
> Psalm 28:7 NKJV

And God was just beginning to use the gifts of those people He surrounded me with.

Our friend Karen wisely asked a key question: "Do you treat many patients with this type of cancer, Doctor?"

"No. I don't see this type of cancer very often," Dr. Collins said hesitantly. "Yours would be my first."

Karen's question probably saved my life by making one thing abundantly clear: not all oncologists are equal! Did I want to partner with a fearful doctor who hadn't treated my type of cancer before, or was it time for a second opinion with a more seasoned professional?

This fight against cancer—with all the questions and decisions—was becoming too much. In one moment I felt the power and strength of God coursing through me, and in the next I felt like collapsing. What I now wanted more than anything was to simply be at home alone with my loving wife Barbi—and for all of this to just go away.

Chapter 3
Finding New Hope

AS I DROVE HOME FROM MY APPOINTMENT WITH DR. COLLINS, I felt an odd sense of aliveness. My life was totally on the line, and I was terrified. But I was also *energized*. I was ready to fight! Absolutely no one or nothing on this earth would keep me from my family, from my wife and our three sons. *Nothing!*

But right next to this dogged determination was paralyzing fear. *What if I don't make it? What if I die and leave my boys fatherless?* Cancer doesn't allow for neutral emotions: every feeling, good and bad, is heightened and punctuated by the risk at hand. This was a kind of intense terror I had never known—and it was purifying.

Purifying? How can cancer be purifying? People die of cancer every day. Fathers leave behind wives and children to fend for themselves. Single mothers leave behind their children. People fight and agonize for years only to eventually succumb to this monstrous disease. The devastation of losing a loved one to cancer brings pain beyond words, beyond imagining. Fighting cancer is serious business. But purifying?

Yes, cancer is deadly serious. And precisely because cancer is deadly serious, it clarifies our thoughts and quickly distills life down to its essential elements. Was I going to shrink and remain in fear, or was I going to fight and take action? Was I going to live or die?

Two Types of Thoughts

On the way home from Dr. Collins', I became aware that really only two types of thoughts mattered now: those that would heal me and those that wouldn't. With my life on the line, the choice was simple: I would eliminate those thoughts that weren't healing thoughts and focus on the ones that were. Putting that decision into practice would be another matter, but deciding how I would fight this battle was an important first step.

With so much at stake, I didn't have the luxury of self-pity. The diagnosis of this life-threatening disease had produced in me a certain energy, and I didn't want to miss this opportunity and waste it on negative thinking. I firmly believe that this energy was a gift from God: He gave me the energy I needed to successfully fight the physical, mental, and emotional demands of the battles that were ahead.

What's the Next Step?

I met Barbi and Karen back at our home in Huntington Beach. Just being in the house produced new waves of tears and fears. This was my home. This is where I lived with my family. The toys and Disney videos scattered about the house; the baseballs and basketballs and trampoline in the backyard; the barbeque where we grilled so many meals; framed pictures from vacations, sports, birthdays, our wedding—this was my life. *And all of this was at stake. I could lose my life, my family, my home....* I felt I could burst into tears at any moment.

On the kitchen counter next to the phone, Karen placed a piece of paper with another oncologist's name and phone number on it. She had listed three numbers—his home, his office, and his cell. "If you want another opinion, Rob, you may want to call Dr. Justice."

I took a deep breath and thanked Karen for the referral. I knew I needed a second opinion, and if I'd had any doubts, those dissolved when Karen reminded me of the significant fact that my type of cancer would be Dr. Collins' first case. But after that pain-filled appointment with a crying doctor, I wasn't up for round two. At least not right this second. Sensing my hesitance, Karen politely said, "Dr. Justice is a customer in [my sister-in-law] Laura's bank, and she told him about you. As a favor to Laura, he's given you his home phone number, which is very unusual for an oncologist to do, but Dr. Justice is a remarkable guy."

Karen's sister-in-law Laura is also a longtime friend of mine, whom I've known since second grade. In 1974, we swam together on the medley relay team that won the "C" league finals for our 11/12 age group. Our families are longtime friends. I greatly appreciated Laura going out of her way on my behalf, but Karen could see that Barbi and I were tired. She didn't press us anymore about calling the new doctor. She gave us both an encouraging hug and left us to rest.

Even though I knew I needed a second opinion about my diagnosis, Dr. Collins' words about my cancer "doubling on the hour" stuck in my head, and I feared we should start treatment right away. Getting a second opinion would require additional appointments and time—time that I might not have to give. I also felt a little uncomfortable about disturbing Dr. Justice, whom I'd never even met, at his home. But Laura and Karen were good friends, so—trusting them and their high opinion of Dr. Justice—I picked up my phone. I didn't wait for business hours: I was desperate. While his phone rang, Barbi and I prayed and asked God for strength and guidance. Our trust in Him was growing—and would continue to grow—in this strange, new world.

> *"Do not fear, for I am with you; do not be dismayed, for I am your God.*
>
> *I will strengthen you and help you; I will uphold you with my righteous right hand."*
>
> God's promise in Isaiah 41:10

The Truth Starts to Sink In

The pleasant woman who answered the phone was Dr. Justice's wife. He wasn't in at the moment, but she assured me she would relay my message to him as soon as he came home later that evening. She patiently took down my name, telephone number, and diagnosis. My fear that I was disturbing the doctor at his home with a "business" call had been quickly dispelled by her calm, soothing manner. I sensed God's care in her kindness. Yet, as hopeful as I felt at that moment, I still had cancer, I was still scared, and what I really wanted to do was to decompress with Barbi and cry.

Barbi's mom had taken our boys to a birthday party so that Barbi and I could be alone together. We had a loft upstairs with a couch, a TV, and a play area for our boys. Barbi and I went up there and collapsed. Interesting that we sought the comfort of our upstairs family room rather than heading to the more formal living room downstairs. Family truly matters....

Purifying Tears

At first we just sat there, crying softly and hugging one another. We had been completely blindsided. *Cancer? How could this be? I'm only thirty-nine! I'm a father of three boys who need me.... My wife needs me.... Barbi's a stay-at-home mom. How will she provide for herself and our sons if I don't survive?... I don't want to die!... I love my wife.... I'm afraid! Oh, God, why is this happening!*

Our emotions spilled out, one after the other, our chests

heaving as we shared each other's pain.

"I don't want to leave you alone," I sobbed.

"You're *not* going to leave me alone!" Barbi cried.

"I feel like… I feel like a failure…."

"You're not a failure, Rob. You're the best thing that's ever happened to me."

"I feel weak. I'm so sorry, honey," I cried.

"You're going to survive this!" Barbi encouraged.

"Austin needs me! Spencie and Colb—I don't want to lose my boys!" I wailed.

As I write these words, even now I'm filled with emotion that makes my heart race. I desperately wanted to be there for Barbi and the boys. I didn't want to stop loving and being loved by them. I didn't want them to be left on their own to fend for themselves, to try to make their own way through this world. Just ten, seven, and five years old, my precious boys were still so innocent. I didn't want them to face the world without me, to grow up without me there to answer all their questions and speak to all their fears, without me there to guide and encourage them.

I felt like a weak man. A failure. What kind of a man leaves his young family? And how hard this was for Barbi! How hard cancer is for the victim's spouse! Not only did Barbi need to process her own fears, but she also needed and wanted to be strong for me, to encourage me, to strengthen me. The supporting spouse can easily feel guilty for thinking about herself and worrying about "What if…." The person with cancer becomes the focus of everyone's attention. The supporting spouse serves as head caregiver and cheerleader—

but who would be Barbi's caregiver and cheerleader? Barbi's fears were just as great as my own, if not greater. If I tapped out, Barbi would be left alone in the ring.

And—the thoughts continued to swirl around me—*do I even have enough life insurance to provide for my family? Now it's too late for me to buy more. I have cancer! How will Barbi support herself? Have I saved enough for my boys to go to college? My God, what had I been doing with my life???* I felt so unprepared.

Barbi remembers that I said to her, "I'm only going to say this once," and I went over with my precious wife all of our financial information and where the records were kept in case I didn't make it.

Admitting these fears, discussing these fears, releasing these fears—all of this was so painful.

The Second Opinion

I didn't realize its significance at the time, but I think one of the healthiest things Barbi and I did in combating this disease was to share all of our deepest, unedited fears as well as the unbridled anger that the diagnosis triggered. And I cannot in good conscience go any further without underscoring how integral God is to this process of raging, grieving, and accepting. Whether or not you believe in Him, if you've been diagnosed with a life-threatening disease, your fears and your anger will sooner or later lead you to a direct confrontation with God. Specifically, you will have to wrestle with whether God is truly an all-knowing, all-powerful, all-loving God... or not.

*"He is wise in heart and mighty in strength—
who has hardened himself against him, and
succeeded?"*

Job 9:4 ESV

The phone rang. It was 10:30 p.m. Barbi and I were exhausted from our day, exhausted by our situation, exhausted from our fear and emotions, exhausted from crying. We were raw. I answered the phone.

"Hello."

"Hello, Rob?"

"Yes, this is Rob. Is this Dr. Justice?"

"Yes, it is—but, please, call me 'friend.'"

I liked the sound of that: *friend*. "OK," I answered somewhat self-consciously.

We discussed my visit to Dr. Collins' office and her initial diagnosis of my cancer, that it was doubling on the hour, and that we needed to begin chemotherapy immediately.

Assuring me that my cancer was not "doubling on the hour," Dr. Justice said that it was far more important to get an accurate diagnosis before beginning treatment. He rattled off several tests that he wanted to perform, and before I knew it, I was signed up for five of them. I remember a chord of fear being struck with the last test mentioned: I would need a spinal tap.

Dr. Collins hadn't ordered any additional testing. Instead, she'd been prepared to begin treatment at once. And while I would have been Dr. Collins' first T-cell lymphoma case, Dr. Justice had treated dozens of cases such as mine because of his affiliation with the USC Norris Cancer Center. There was a vast difference between the two doctors' experience with cancer and the attendant confidence they inspired—or didn't. I was seeing very clearly that *not all doctors are created equal* when it comes to tackling a particular disease. That's one reason why it is *extremely important to get a second opinion.*

In Dr. Collins' office I had felt great fear. In her mind, the science of the lymphoma had already condemned me, and when I'd asked about my prognosis, she'd cried. I was her first T-cell lymphoma case, and I don't know who was more afraid—the doctor or me! We were both in this for the first time, and neither one of us knew how best to treat this cancer.

But one thing was clear to me: God had allowed that visit to Dr. Collins' to drive me to my knees in desperation. God overwhelmed my ability to self-manage and allowed the fear of Dr. Collins to be evident in her tears. Dr. Collins may have been the one Dr. Barnes referred me to, but God had other plans. He used my appointment with Dr. Collins to graciously move me to the point where the only thing I could do was pray, surrendering my disease and myself to Him. It seemed clear that God was asking me to trust Him. And then, when I—in desperation—had humbled myself and, in prayer, entrusted myself to God, how quickly He responded!

> *"LORD, hear my prayer, listen to my cry for mercy;*
> *in your faithfulness and righteousness come to*
> *my relief."*
>
> Psalm 143:1

Within minutes of getting home from my disheartening appointment with Dr. Collins, my friend Karen gave me the card of a doctor who *happens* to be an expert in my particular cancer, with his home phone number, that was secured by my childhood friend Laura, who *happens* to be his private banker. *Coincidence?? Luck??* Perhaps.

My belief, however, is that when you open your heart to God and put your trust in Him, you begin to realize that the whole world is under His absolute control and that no one is out of His reach when He wants to connect you with someone important. And God knows just which friends, friends of friends, relatives, co-workers, and/or acquaintances can best help you. I'm very grateful that Karen and Laura were available to help me when God nudged them. What a blessing!

And isn't evidence of God everywhere? When you look at your son or daughter or loved one, do you really believe that this love is the product of complete randomness played out on a godless planet? Or can you allow for, in whatever form, the presence of divinity, of a Creator who created you with love? We may have abandoned God, but that doesn't mean that God has abandoned us. And God is anxious to renew His relationship with you and to strengthen you—if you'll allow Him. But you must also take action. Simply put:

> *"Humble yourselves before the Lord,*
> *and he will lift you up."*
>
> James 4:10

I humbled myself, I called on the Lord, and God led me—using my friends—to a new doctor and fresh hope.

"Rob, there are two things you need to know about T-cell lymphoma," Dr. Justice told me. "One, you're curable. And, two, you're in recovery right now."

Once again, I began to cry. But these tears were different.

Chapter 4
Telling the Kids

"WHAT DO WE TELL OUR CHILDREN?" MY WIFE HAD ASKED.
In response, Dr. Collins cried.

Cancer is serious business.

So, what would we tell our children? If you're in this situation, what will you tell your children? We had no clue—and neither had Dr. Collins. What we did know was that we needed help from someone stronger than we were. Barbi and I needed God's wisdom, God's strength, and God's guidance to face our enemy head-on and fight this battle—and we'd be fighting on many fronts. We would fight to prepare ourselves for the battle. We would fight the cancer itself with treatment and prayer. We would fight the battle of confronting fears—my fear of losing loved ones and my loved ones' fear of losing me. We would fight to keep life happening—and happening as smoothly as possible. After all, with or without cancer, I'm still a husband. With or without cancer, I'm still Dad. I can't just check out. I needed to be strong for Barbi and for my three boys—and I needed help.

For me, one blessing of cancer was apparent right away in that it quickly drove me to my knees to ask for God's help, but the cancer ultimately had me on my feet as I cried out: "This cancer is not bigger than God, and we will not run from it in fear!"

Wow! Where did that proclamation come from! Some people might say it was prompted by adrenaline and desperation. They would say I reacted the way a mother does when she lifts a car off of her child who is trapped underneath. I was scared, to be sure, but that fear drove me to declare my faith more boldly than I ever had: "THIS CANCER IS *NOT* BIGGER THAN GOD! " I was pissed off! I wasn't dead yet, and there was no way in hell that I was going to give in to the fear of f-ing cancer and leave my boys fatherless and my wife quivering and beaten. I was furious! Clearly—and this is another blessing of cancer—that disease unleashed a lion that I never knew was inside me.

Again, where did this strength come from? I've always seen myself as a rather mild-mannered guy, not particularly bold or self-confident. I would not characterize myself as a fighter. But Barbi fights for what she believes in, and I've always admired her strength. Me? I prefer to talk tough from the sidelines and stew when I don't get my way. But not this time! This time was different. This time *I* was different.

This time, when the bully stepped up in front of me, I called him out. Cancer awakened the lion within me, and I was determined to fight back, for me and for my family. *But what exactly do I do to marshal the energy behind this roar?*

When you found out about your cancer, you may have exploded with a similar roar either internally or, as I did, out loud. Or perhaps you've been so terrified of what's coming that you've numbed yourself into a catatonic state or, worse, you've accepted cancer as a death sentence and have basically given up. Experiencing all these emotions is normal, I think, but whatever you're feeling right now, know that there is One who is not afraid of your cancer and who is in fact very able to help you confront it. I'm talking about the all-knowing, all-powerful, all-loving Creator of the universe, your Father God.

When I sat in Dr. Collins' office, learned about my cancer, and was essentially told to prepare our kids for the worst, God gave me a far different admonition: "Prepare your kids to see your best." How? By trusting in Him and in His unlimited power.

> *"Behold, I am the LORD, the God of all flesh.*
>
> *Is there anything too hard for Me?"*
>
> Jeremiah 32:27 NKJV

If you're already planning your own funeral, don't be so quick to write yourself off. God may have a different design for you. After all, as the Scripture says, nothing is too hard for God—and that includes beating cancer.

A Solid Plan

Even before I had specific ideas, I knew for sure that just as Barbi and I needed God's help to fight this fight, we needed His help in determining how best to tell our boys. So Barbi and I prayed a lot. As we prayed, God prompted us to consult with some close friends, a few relatives, and our pastor. The advice we received led us to a solid plan we could get behind: *Be honest with the children and invite them into the process.*

Barbi and I continued to pray about our battle against cancer, but we also started asking God to give us the strength to be honest and confident as we told the boys about my cancer. Our strategy was to speak positively about the treatment and talk briefly about its possible side effects.

"Boys, Mom and I have something to tell you," I began. "You know I've been around the house a lot this last week and not going into work. I've been getting tests done to find out what's been going on with my rib and underneath my arm." The boys knew about my rib. They thought it was pretty funny that their dad broke his rib with a sneeze.

"Isn't that what we go to the Jacuzzi for?" asked Spencer. For several weeks after I ingloriously broke my rib, the boys and I would walk down to the community Jacuzzi after dinner and soak. The warm water felt good and relieved some of the pain.

"Yes, Spencer, that's right. But the doctor found something else."

"Daddy has curable lymphoma," Barbi said. The word *curable* had come to us when we talked with Dr. Justice. We were going after *cure*. That was the word Dr. Justice had used, and that was the vision he wanted to plant in my head: *cure*. Not survival, but *cure*. Much of today's thought in cancer circles is about "surviving with cancer," and some doctors are reluctant to get a patient's hopes up by discussing a cure when certain statistics may not be as hopeful. I understand that approach, but to me that's akin to playing prevent defense in a football game. Yeah, it can work; it's one strategy. My goal and my doctor's approach called for a mindset of beating the opponent. We were not after survival; we were after *cure*.

"What's that?" asked Austin, our oldest son.

"Lymphoma is a type of cancer that infects the lymph nodes in your body," I said. "I'll need to take medicine, which is called chemotherapy, to help get rid of the lymphoma. The chemotherapy is the medicine that will cure me."

So far, so good. We're telling the truth; no fibs. Barbi and I are holding up OK, and the boys are quietly processing the news. No need to go into the type of blood disorder I had. Just cover the basics.

Here Come the Questions

"In the coming weeks we'll be looking for several things that will tell us the medicine is working," Barbi explained. "One of them is that Dad's hair will start to fall out."

The boys looked surprised.

"Daddy's going to be bald?" asked Colby. His nose scrunched up as he smiled sheepishly at the thought of his father losing his hair. *My God,* I thought to myself, *Colby is so innocent, and I never want to betray his trust.* I found myself filled with an even greater resolve to survive.

Our oldest son was connecting the dots. "Is Dad going to be OK?" Austin asked. "Don't people die from cancer?"

Uh-oh! There it was. The dreaded question I'd known would come. And it may be the very question you're facing right now. All the fear seems to come down to just one question: "Don't people die from cancer?" *Give me words, Lord.*

"Yes, Austin. Cancer is serious, and some people do die. But the type of cancer I have is curable," I said. I knew it was important to be honest, to acknowledge Austin's fear, but also to clearly state that what I had was curable. And not wanting to lie to Austin, I realized that if I told him it was curable (which it was), then I myself needed to believe that I was curable. There was no benefit in discussing statistics or survival rates. Just the big picture. How would discussing survival statistics help anything? The truth is, T-cell lymphoma does have a cure rate.

Austin quietly processed the information.

"Dad's going to be OK," Barbi assured him.

"I'm going to be fine, boys." In truth, I was beginning to get a bit wobbly. "I'm going to be fine, but I'm going to need your help, and so is Mom. One of the side effects of the medicine I'll get during chemotherapy—besides losing my hair—is that I may not be feeling well all the time. We're all going to need to help out around the house and do our homework without complaining, and there may be times when I'm not able to wrestle as much."

Groans all around.

The boys were OK with the homework and the chores, but

missing out on wrestling was another matter. Our wrestling was a nightly ritual, and we'd wrestle until someone cried or got hurt. Then Mom would come upstairs and demand that we stop. Poor Barbi. She could never understand why, with at least one "injury" per night guaranteed, the boys continued to want to wrestle with their father night after night.

"We want you to know that lymphoma is serious, but it is curable," I said. "Do you have any more questions for me or Mom?"

"Are you still going to be able to play baseball with me?" asked Spencer.

"Yes, Spencer. I'll still be able to play baseball with you. And swim and play roller hockey too."

"Are you still going to coach my team?" asked Colby.

"Yes, Colby. I will still be your coach."

The boys seemed OK with everything and were starting to get restless. This was usually the segue into wrestling, which we ultimately did, but not until we first said a prayer. Barbi led: "Dear Lord, thank You for the doctors and for the medicine that will help cure Daddy. We pray that we can all work together and that you will bless our family with good health. And we pray that Daddy's hair will fall out so we know the medicine is working."

Colby snickered.... Spencer seemed ready to move on.... And I couldn't quite read Austin. This experience would test the boys' faith as much as it would test mine.

Barbi and I both felt it was important for our sons to see us being candid, prayerful, and strong, and we didn't want them to be blindsided by side effects that might otherwise scare them. But was I being honest enough about the downside of my cancer, about the cure rate? What if your cancer is more serious than mine? Perhaps you have ovarian or brain cancer, or are facing life-and-death surgery, or have much, much lower survival rates. How do you approach your children in these circumstances?

Perhaps the conversation with my sons would have been different if my cancer had been that severe, but I felt the conversation was appropriate to my circumstances. Was I in denial about the seriousness of my circumstances—of my cancer—when I spoke to my sons? Fair question, but I would answer that there is more than one way of navigating through cancer, no matter its severity. The best guideline Barbi and I found was simply to consider—each step of the way—what sort of example we wanted to be for our family and ask God to help us be that kind of example. We chose not to say, "Cancer has a 75% chance of taking my life, so don't get your hopes up!" Sometimes in an attempt to present a "balanced" view, we spend so much time on the negatives that we lose energy for the positives. In reality, as long as there was a cure rate, the odds were fairly meaningless. Barbi and I chose to give our boys the positive example of fighting the battle while resting in the truth that God will provide no matter what the outcome.

Again, my path is only one possible way, and by God's grace, this approach worked for my family and me. I didn't want to give cancer a chance, and I certainly didn't want to give it a voice. I wanted to beat the shit out of it.

Physical Activity, Emotional Reassurance

I believed that continuing to be physically active would further assure my sons that Dad's medicine was working and would address any unspoken fears and anxieties they may have had. Actions do speak louder than words.

While I have always enjoyed playing sports, what I really appreciated during my battle with cancer were these underlying reasons why sports are so great:

- Being active is a declaration of life, and it reaffirmed to my boys—and to me—that I was alive.

- Being involved in sports demonstrated that I was physically strong.

- Physical activity was a great way to connect with my sons—and it was fun!

- A sports-playing dad is a living dad, not a dying one, so my activity gave my sons emotional reassurance that I was fighting to win.

- Exercise has always stimulated my mental as well as my physical well-being.

- Exercise is a healthy way to channel the negative energy produced by the fear of cancer and the fear of dying into the positive energy of living.

- Exercise took power away from cancer and gave it back to me.

This kind of healthy activity gave cancer a new face.

"The New Face of Cancer"

Each year the weekend after Memorial Day weekend (when temperatures rose and prices dropped), we would take a family vacation at the Shadow Mountain Resort in Palm Desert with our friends the Godfreys and their three sons. We would rent a two-bedroom condo right on a huge greenbelt and adjacent to an enormous (advertised as the largest in the desert) figure-8 pool. That condo was a wonderful madhouse. We adults took the two bedrooms, and the six boys all slept in the living room in sleeping bags on the pull-out couches and the floor. Our days were filled with tennis, golf, swimming, volleyball, baseball, and Jacuzziing. The boys were able to run off and have an adventure, while we all grabbed a moment or or two of adult time, had a glass of wine, and relaxed. For a few days I could forget that I had stage 4 cancer.

One day after I'd been throwing the boys up in the air in the pool for what seemed like half the day—"Daddy, Daddy, throw me up again, pleeease!"—Barbi coined a term for me. Seeing how invigorated I was and how happily the kids were splashing around, she dubbed the Raban approach to healing "the new face of cancer." I instantly took that phrase to heart. Cancer had a new face because, at least for me, it wasn't the face of someone defeated by circumstances. God had blessed me with a strength I had no right to expect in the middle of a rigorous chemo regimen. And to be physically active in the pool with my sons and enjoying the warmth of the sun was so life affirming. "The new face of cancer" was an empowering term. I really liked it—and I definitely wanted to be that guy! I pray that you will want to be "the new face of cancer" in your own personal way.

A Real-Life Example

What I found with cancer is that it gives you a chance to show your family—and yourself—the true meaning of faith. The diagnosis of cancer and its subsequent treatment are opportunities to demonstrate trusting your heavenly Father, praying, submitting to God's will, and asking for His help. Children watch us, and they see the path they can walk when they face their own obstacles. Your commitment to fight your cancer and live life to the fullest, even when you're unsure of the outcome, is an unmistakable demonstration of faith in the God for whom nothing is impossible. You don't know the outcome, but you keep fighting. That's the picture of faith I wanted to model for my sons.

> *"The LORD is my light and my salvation;*
>   *Whom shall I fear?*
>
> *The LORD is the strength of my life;*
>   *Of whom shall I be afraid?"*
>
> Psalm 27:1 NKJV

Your children are watching how you handle this adversity. What sort of example will you be for them?

Chapter 5
Dreams That Matter

I FIRST MET DR. JUSTICE IN PERSON ON MONDAY, MARCH 25,
2002. He asked that I be his last appointment of the day so
that he could spend uninterrupted time with me. I felt very
fortunate to be able to see this doctor.

Dr. Justice was the director of the Fountain Valley Regional
Cancer Center, a facility affiliated with the USC Norris Cancer
Center where he was a clinical professor. He was president of
the American Cancer Society Orange County division and sat
on the board of directors for the American Cancer Society of
California and other notable organizations. Dr. Justice was the
real deal, and I was anxious to meet him in person. Barbi, our
friend Karen, and I sat in the warmly furnished reception area
waiting to be called. A nurse opened a door to the examination
rooms and invited us back to Dr. Justice's office....

I had been praying for God to lead me to the best doctor to
treat my cancer, and I wanted to believe that Dr. Justice was

the one. He had been so friendly on the phone when we spoke, and he had sounded confident that my cancer was curable. As much as I wanted to believe that I could beat cancer, I also wanted to be sure that Dr. Justice was the doctor God had in mind for me. As we waited for him in his office, I was looking for a sign that he was the right doctor for me. I noticed a Bible on his desk and thought to myself, *That's a good sign.* I also noticed a diploma from USC on the wall. A fellow Trojan! Another good sign. And at just that moment, Dr. Justice ambled in looking like a diminutive Santa Claus with a round belly, balding head, sparkling eyes, and a demeanor that said, "We don't shake hands here; we hug."

"Dr. J"—as his patients call him—was just as warm in person as he had been on the phone. When I asked Dr. J about the Bible on his desk, he said that he is a Christian and that he goes to Mariners, a church not too far from St. Andrews Presbyterian where I attended at the time. He was also in a men's Bible study that met on Tuesday nights. As far as signs go, God was laying them out for me: I was also in a men's Bible study, and we also met on Tuesday nights. As we talked, Dr. J shared that some people who had the same cancer I had would not survive, and he reaffirmed how important exercising faith would be to my healing. Cancer is not bigger than God, and here I had a doctor who shared and strengthened my belief. His office was quite a change from the fearful environment of Dr. Collins' office!

These were important signs that helped me feel more comfortable about choosing Dr. Justice, but there was one more sign that grabbed my heart with a jolt, and in that moment I knew Dr. J was truly the doctor God planned to use for my treatment and cure. On the wall hung a copy of Winslow Homer's famous painting *Breezin' Up*, a picture of a father wordlessly passing on his knowledge of life and the sea to his three young sons as the four of them sailed in a small boat on the Eastern Seaboard. It is my favorite picture, meaningful because, among other reasons, I am also the father of three boys.

In the painting, the sea is a little rough, but the middle son nevertheless has ventured outside the cockpit and is lying across the bow, holding on tightly, clearly testing his boundaries. The father's countenance is calm and reassuring. The oldest son has hiked out on the stern of the boat to man the tiller, modeling the way of responsibility for his brothers, while the youngest son is positioned safely in the cockpit, pushing his boundary mildly as he sits on the gunnel rounding the perimeter of cockpit, content with his own thoughts and place. Despite the rough waters, the boys are secure in their father's presence. It's a wonderful painting—and it's one that I have hanging prominently on the wall in my office at home. Call it coincidence, call it luck, call it what you will, but I can tell you that I call the appearance of that painting in Dr. J's office "answered prayer."

To me it was clear that God had chosen Dr. Justice to be my doctor.

"Being Accurate"

Dr. Justice had ordered a battery of tests to be run immediately. He did not accept the preliminary diagnosis that my cancer was doubling on the hour and that we needed to start chemo immediately.

"Being accurate is more important than being fast," Dr. J countered. "I want the best minds in the country to look at your slides to determine exactly what you have so we can prescribe the most effective treatment." (Due to Dr. J's affiliation with USC, a renowned pathologist at the Keck School of Medicine would help with my evaluation.)

I liked Dr. J's confidence, and there was no question that he was confident in his ability to treat cancer. His board affiliations and awards were also reassuring. But it was Dr. J's warmth and his faith in God as the ultimate Healer that really drew me to him.

I liked being on Dr. J's team! I was determined to be the kind of cooperative, faithful patient this good doctor wanted. I totally bought into Dr. J's program, which included "not searching the internet and trying the blueberry cure or some other such nonsense." Avoiding potential distractions was crucial, and Dr. J was very direct: "When you're on my team, I want you to follow my program. Let me be the expert."

One part of the program that was primarily my responsibility was to maintain my weight. Chemotherapy is notorious for whittling away at the patient's body, leaving him or her vulnerable to infection, pneumonia, and a host of other maladies. Dr. J wanted me to eat anything that would keep my weight on: "I don't care if you have to eat McDonald's Big Macs and fries to keep the weight on. Just do it."

I protested that I have high cholesterol. Dr. J chuckled, "You've got bigger problems than your cholesterol right now. Let's just confirm your diagnosis first, and then we'll worry about your diet."

Among my tests would be a bone marrow biopsy, a nuclear PET scan, a CT scan with contrast, a bone scan, an echocardiogram to measure the strength of my heart (so they would know how much chemo they could blast me with), and a spinal tap. Basically, I would have a test a day. I was anxious about the week ahead, so I did the best thing I could: I gave this fear to God.

God Prepares Me: Dream #1

Before going to bed on Sunday night, Barbi and I prayed for restful sleep and for peace despite the uncertainty of what lay ahead. We knew that the keys to fighting my cancer would be not only my mental strength, physical strength, diet, and exercise program, but also the quality of my rest.

I placed a couple of T-shirts on my nightstand and a terry cloth towel underneath me to absorb the sweat that would come during my sleep. A telltale sign of lymphoma is night sweats, and I was sweating through two to three T-shirts a night. As Barbi said a prayer for me, inviting God into our healing, I began to relax, and soon I drifted off to sleep.

That evening God blessed me with a powerful dream. It was a short dream, but a very powerful one....

My three sons were swimming in the ocean. I was hovering in the sky above, looking down on them. It was a sunny day, and for some reason we were at the beach in Malibu. We'd driven through Malibu so I knew what it looked like, but I'd never been to the beach in Malibu. (We normally just went to the beach in Huntington where we live.) In my dream the water at Malibu was a shimmering greenish blue, and the cliffs were rocky and bare. There was an outline of houses along the shore, and people I didn't know were lying here and there on the sand. I began to ascend higher, and my boys became smaller. I was leaving my sons!

Stop! I don't want to go higher! I don't want to leave my boys! And like the parent filled with the strength to lift a car off of his trapped child, I bolted back to earth—back to my sons—in an adrenaline-powered dive toward the water below. Nothing would keep me from the boys I loved. They needed me!

We've all had dreams where we were being pursued by a bad guy from whom we couldn't escape, or we were in a fight where we couldn't throw a punch with any power, as if we were in a vat of glue and all of our actions were in slow motion. This dream was the opposite of that. Nothing was constraining me! This dream filled me with so much power. I felt strong! My love for my sons, their love for me, my fear of not being there for them, my profound desire to be there for them—the confluence of fear, desire, and love compelled me to take action. Decisive action! My faith lived out! In a flash I dived down and rescued my sons. No sticky glue in this dream was going to hold me back!

I awoke from that dream with a steely, lock-jawed

determination that I would survive this cancer. I would be there for my family.

God showed me in my dream that I had the will, the strength, and the capacity to live on. When I woke on that first morning of testing, I was energized and ready to go. What an incredible gift the Lord had given me! He had replaced my fear with strength and my doubt, with hope.

God Prepares Me: Dream #2

The very next night I had another dream, far different from the one the night before, but equally powerful....

I was riding along in a golf cart with my son Austin. It was a gorgeous sunny day, one of those ideal days where you feel neither hot nor cold. I felt relaxed, as if I were watching a summertime evening baseball game where nothing's required of you but to sit, watch, and enjoy. I felt peaceful. Ahh, peace. I hadn't felt that in a while!

Austin and I were sitting side by side, dressed comfortably in our golf shirts and Bermuda shorts. I was driving the cart, and we passed several holes. Rather than pushing to get to a particular hole, we were just enjoying the ride. And while the ride in the golf cart wasn't very bumpy, it wasn't particularly smooth either. There were ups and downs, but Austin and I managed them without fear or discomfort. I saw a few other people on the course, but they took no notice of Austin and me. They seemed part of the background, like the green grass and trees laid out before us. There were no burdens on Austin or me to be social or behave according to golf's protocol. We just drove our cart unfettered as if we had the entire course to ourselves.

I was keenly aware of the beauty of the hilly course. As we drove the golf cart, though, we went over patches of grass that were worn and in need of reseeding, but these dry spots didn't detract from the course's beauty. These imperfect spots were simply part of the course. The beauty of the course lay not in the kind of pristine nature one might associate with Augusta or Pebble Beach, but rather in the rich feeling of being connected with my son, playing golf with him on a warm, sunny day, and not having a care in the world. The beauty of the course, therefore, was really not the beauty of the course, but rather the beauty of the easy, carefree moment.

This description suggests it was a rather ordinary dream, but it has been seared in my mind for these last ten years. During the week of testing that it preceded and the uncertainty of the cancer journey ahead, that dream offered remarkable comfort.

The Gift of Peace

What stood out most in this dream was my complete lack of concern for my circumstances. There was no throbbing "Oh, I've got cancer" ache resonating in my gut. No shiver of fear that I might not make it. Just a feeling of hope. And, although at the time getting Austin to do his homework was always a challenge, I felt no stabs of "We've got to get back and do your homework" anxiety. Instead, the dream brought a feeling of contentment in the present moment and a feeling of hope for the future.

The curious thing is that, in the dream, Austin and I never did stop at a hole. We never hit a drive, sank a putt, or chipped out of a sand trap. In fact, we never even swung a club. We were observers, and we simply drove across the holes of a hilly golf course with its dirt patches and the day's perfect weather. So why did God allow me this dream, this feeling of contentment—and what exactly did it mean?

I find it significant that Austin was the only other family member in my dream. Austin is my firstborn and, as such, the first in line to inherit my role as patriarch of the family. In biblical times, the firstborn son received a double inheritance from his father, so he would have the resources both to carry on the family business and to serve in the role of patriarch by, for instance, hosting family gatherings. Being the firstborn, Austin received a lot of attention from doting grandparents and from his expectant parents who had so much hope and anticipation about their firstborn. One's firstborn is special.

So, in terms of the dream, Austin carried both my hope for the future and the Raban family name for generations to come. As my oldest son, Austin was positioned to lead his brothers and be the example to follow should something happen to me. Austin is also the first to resist my parenting, challenge my discipline and say no to me, as all children eventually do, so at times we were in conflict. And yet here we were, in this dream, completely and comfortably connected. No conflicts, no disagreements, no discord. Just peace.

As I drove the golf cart, I felt no sense of urgency, no pull from a destination we needed to reach or a place we needed to find, no time schedule that needed to be kept. I wasn't anxious about any conversation we needed to have, any topics we needed to discuss or plans we needed to make. We didn't talk about his baseball team or my work, about chores undone or run-ins with his brothers. There were no dogs to walk, no poop to pick up, no groceries to buy, no food to cook, no bills to pay, no lawns to mow, no cars to wash, no doctor appointments to go to, no cancer to fight, no challenges to face. *We took a break.*

What made this dream truly remarkable was not what the dream was about, but what it *wasn't* about. At this particular point in time, when I was feeling the weight of the world on my shoulders, God gifted me with a dream of emotional weightlessness. How was it possible to feel so carefree when my fight against cancer lay before me—with a myriad of scans, biopsies, chemotherapy, and a spinal tap no less! The Bible talks about the peace God gives that "surpasses all understanding," and this dream brought me that kind of peace. God was comforting me for the journey to come, telling me that it would be bumpy and hilly, that there would be dry patches along the way, but that there would also be remarkable beauty and great peace.

> *"You will keep him in perfect peace,*
> *Whose mind is stayed on You,*
> *Because he trusts in You."*
>
> Isaiah 26:3 NKJV

Eternal Words of Truth

When I awoke in the morning, I felt deeply rested and comfortable rather than anxious and restless about the battery of tests that would soon begin. Instead of having a knot in my stomach, I enjoyed a divine peace in the blessed aftermath of my extraordinary dreams. When Barbi woke, she told me that she, too, had slept very well. God had given both of us the gift of rest, and we were grateful.

God was telling me that I did not need to fear my cancer journey. A dream of power followed by a dream of peace—what better gifts could God have given me in preparation for the week ahead? Imagine the impact on your ability to face cancer—or any other adversity, for that matter—when you wake up without fear and doubt in your heart, but with strength and hope.

Imagine that.

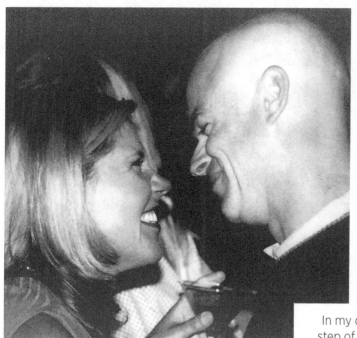

In my corner every
step of the way, my
best friend and love of
my life — Barbi.

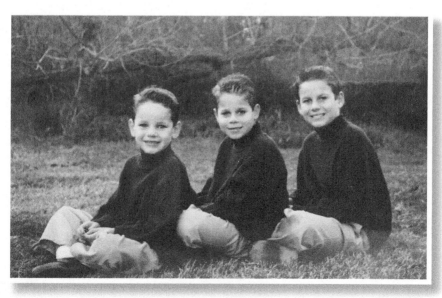

My three sons, Austin, Spencer and Colby.

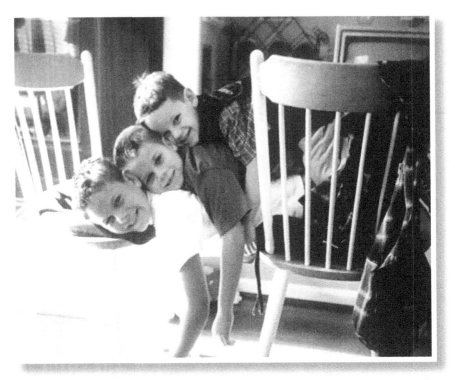

Three reasons why I was willing to do
anything to fight and survive!!

Spencer, Colby and
Austin with our dog Pax

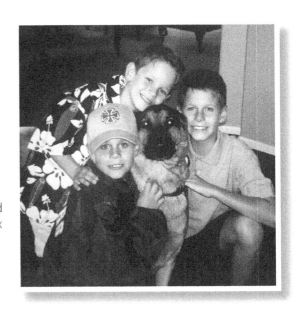

Little League Opening Day
With Barbi, Colby,
Spencer and Austin
Three weeks before
I was diagnosed

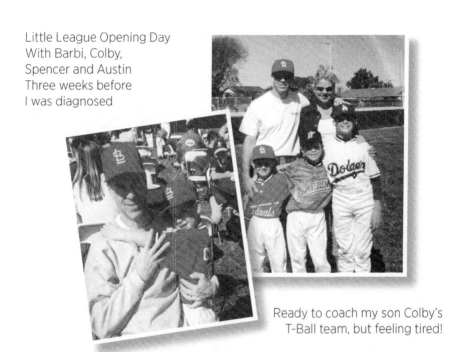

Ready to coach my son Colby's
T-Ball team, but feeling tired!

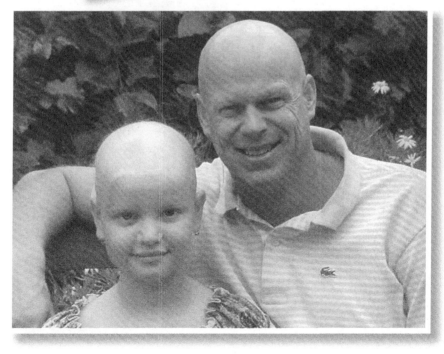

With my friend Karina who was
courageously battling Leukemia at age 7.

Prayer Warriors — my sister, Marci, and my mom Harlene

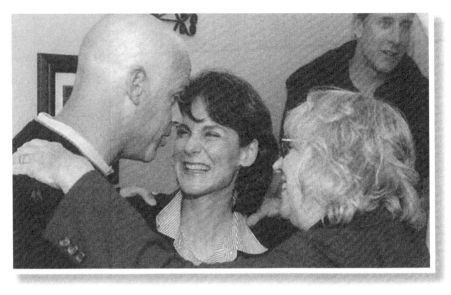

My dad, Bob Raban, who fought prostate cancer at the same time I was undergoing chemo.

(I'm pictured here a few years later when I had hair again!)

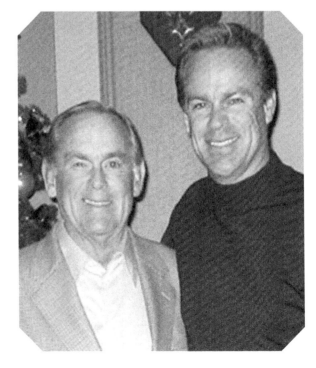

With Randy Clark,
my best man and
lifelong friend
from 2nd grade.

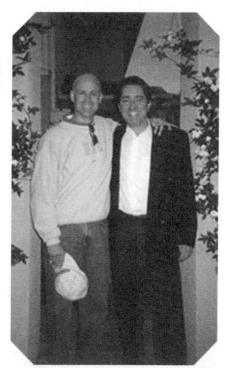

With David Casey, another
lifelong friend from 2nd Grade
planning matters I was forced to
deal with when my grandfather died
two months into my chemotherapy.

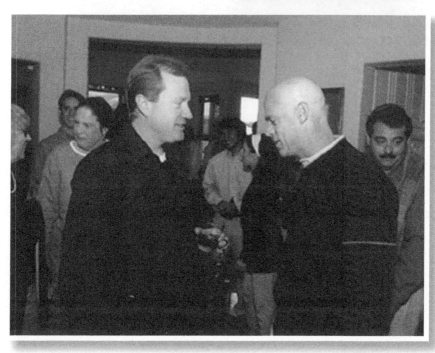

With Karen Koeller, who accompanied me to my doctors'
appointments, and her husband, Charlie, another close
friend from grade school and the associate pastor of our
church. Charlie and Karen were an invaluable source of
love and support each step of the way.

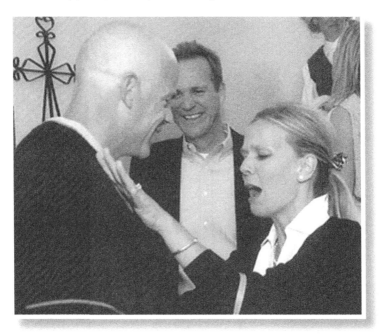

Laughing with my
childhood friend Laura
who introduced me
to Dr. Justice, and his
second opinion saved
my life. Years later
Laura succumbed to
Ovarian cancer after a
Herculean battle.

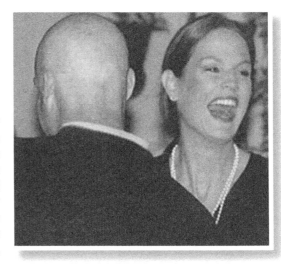

My co-workers at Industrial Valco shaved their heads in support for me! Pictured in the second row, far left, is my 86 year old grandfather 'Nick' who would pass on a few weeks after this photo was taken, adding the additional responsibility of managing the family business while undergoing chemo. Praise God I was not alone!

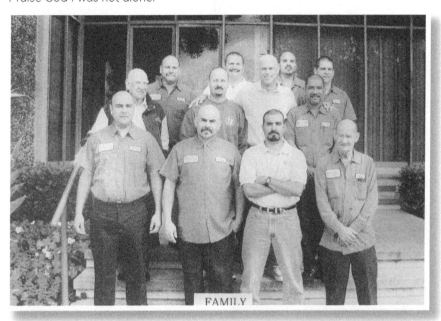

FAMILY

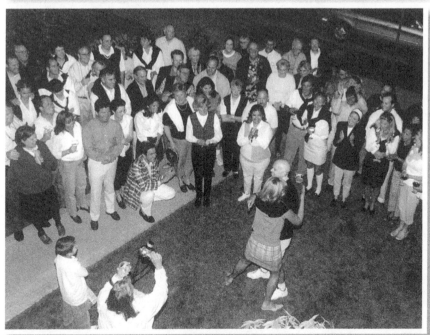

Saying thanks to friends and family who gave so much to Barbi and me!

My weekend basketball buddies kidnapped my shoe, named him "Lefty," and sent me 'ransom' photos from around the country.

Rob Rabån
6572 Brentwood Drive
Huntington Beach, California 92648

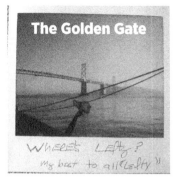

The Golden Gate

Where's Lefty? my best to all "Lefty"

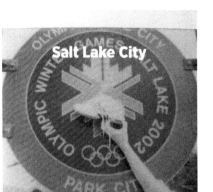

Salt Lake City

You never took me anywhere "Lefty"

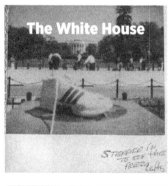

The White House

Stepped in to see the prez..."Lefty"

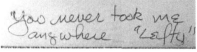
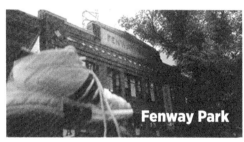

Fenway Park

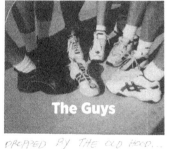

The Guys

Dropped by the old hood... still got my game...and you

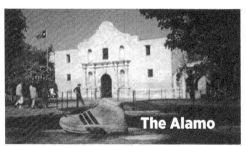

The Alamo

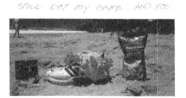

Lefty took an amazing journey--and my heart along with him!

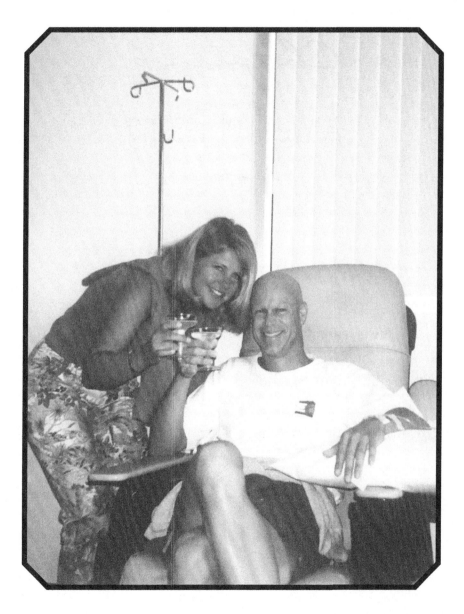

Cheers! Celebrating with Barbi on the last day of chemo!

Chapter 6

A Week of Testing

REFRESHED AND STRENGTHENED BY DREAMS OF PEACE AND power, I was ready to begin working on my recovery. It would be a busy first week, with Dr. Justice ordering the following tests to confirm my diagnosis:

Tuesday	9:15 a.m.	Echocardiogram
Wednesday	12:30 p.m.	Nuclear PET Scan (Position Emission Tomography)
Thursday	8:30 a.m.	Abdominal/Pelvic CT Scan (Computed Tomography)
Friday	10:30 a.m.	Spinal Tap
Friday	4:30 p.m.	Bone Marrow Aspiration (Conscious Sedation)

Tuesday at 9:15 a.m. – Echocardiogram

An echocardiogram measures the strength of your heart. High frequency, ultrasonic sound waves are transmitted by a wand-like device, called a transducer, to your heart. The sound waves bounce off your heart and through your tissues and produce an "echo" of reflected waves that can be recorded through the transducer and sent to a computer for analysis. The movement of the heart and the echoing of the sound waves enable images to be taken of the heart (Cancer.net). This test— basically an ultrasound of the heart—is routinely prescribed in order to check for preexisting heart conditions before a person begins chemotherapy. Heart damage is a possible side effect of some chemo drugs and can lead to arrhythmias, a weakening of the heart, or congestive heart failure. Basically, Dr. Justice ordered the test to find out how much chemo he could blast me without causing problems elsewhere. *Great.*

On Tuesday morning Barbi and I drove down to Newport Heart, a testing clinic in Newport Beach, for our 9:15 appointment. We checked in at the front desk and were given some forms to fill out. We sat down on a comfortable couch and began to fill in the information requested when one of Barbi's friends, Debbie, walked into the room.

One of the blessings of being in a church family is the support of friends in times of need. Barbi and I are Christians, and at the time Barbi was in a Bible study with eight other women, all of whom were praying for me. When Debbie met us at the clinic to offer moral support and her prayers, we realized that having a friend at some appointments is a real blessing. Friends like Debbie remind you that you're not alone, that someone cares about you, and that there's another world outside the doctor's office and beyond your illness. Barbi and I were comforted by Debbie's presence: she helped make the environment significantly less alien.

Soon after I finished filling out the forms, Amy, the nurse technician, called me back to the testing room and had me take off my shirt. I was asked to lie down on my side with my upper body exposed. She applied a small amount of gel to my chest and then moved the transducer around, allowing the sound waves and heart echo to paint its picture. The test was totally painless and took only a few minutes.

Although I wasn't to get the full report for a few days, Amy told me that I "did well" on my test. She said my heart was "very strong" and at the "upper highest level of normal." Even if I lost 10% of my heart capacity from the chemo, I would still be in "normal" range. Thirsting for any good news, I was grateful that Amy told me I had a strong heart. I appreciated the encouragement—and I'd made it through my first test. Praise God!

Wednesday at 12:30 p.m. – PET Scan

PET stands for "Positron Emission Tomography," and this procedure uses nuclear medicine to produce three-dimensional images of what's going on in your body. My dog, Pax, joined me at this appointment. Now, I can be a little slow on the uptake sometimes, but not until I wrote this chapter did I realize the beauty of taking my *pet* Pax—whose name means "peace"—to the *PET* scan appointment. God was providing a pet for my PET. It was His little wink that said, "Don't worry, Rob. Be at peace. I'm watching out for you."

We had recently adopted Pax, a beautiful German shepherd, from a guide dog school for the blind. Pax was more interested in discovering the world around him than paying attention to his "blind" trainers, so Pax was dismissed from training and made available for adoption. We'd had Pax for about six months at the time my testing began, yet I felt that this beautiful and powerful dog somehow knew something was wrong with me. Pax would look at me with canine compassion and then lick my face, almost as if he were taking care of a puppy in need. As we pulled into the parking lot before my test, Pax gave me a reassuring lick on the cheek.

After filling out more forms and providing my insurance information, I was taken back to a quiet room with an oversized, padded La-Z-Boy chair, low lighting, warm, natural colors, and a Zen water fountain to relax me. I sat down in the La-Z-Boy, and the nurse technician checked my glucose with a finger prick. Then she put an IV in the back of my left hand. Next, a dose of radioactive glucose was injected through my IV. The radioactivity is so powerful that the vial containing it is housed in a half-inch-thick cylinder of tungsten steel. The nurse held the tungsten housing and depressed the plunger so as to avoid direct contact with the radioactive vial. I was then instructed to lie back and relax for forty-five minutes;

I was not to talk or move. No problem there! You give me forty-five minutes of uninterrupted time to nap and, cancer or no cancer, I'm in!

After those forty-five minutes, I was taken into the PET scan room, asked to lie down on a narrow bed, covered with a warm blanket, and told to stretch my hands over my head. A big barrel encircled the lower half of the bed and started making a whizzing sound. The bed slowly moved farther into the barrel, inch by inch, as pictures of my internal organs were taken. I was again instructed not to move during the forty-five minutes of the test. Classical music was playing, and I took advantage of another forty-five minutes of naptime and went back to sleep.

While I napped, *the* radioactive glucose was rapidly synthesized by highly metabolic cancer cells. The PET scan shows images of this synthesis and pinpoints hot spots of activity. From this, doctors can see the location of the cancer and whether it has spread to other organs. They can also determine the treatment needed to eradicate the cancer.

I felt fine after the test. Relaxed, a little groggy, but OK. I was told to drink a lot of water to help move along the radioactive glucose that was still in my system. I was assured it would be gone in twenty-four hours, but as a precaution, I was asked to avoid pregnant women and children five years old and younger because of the radioactivity still coursing through my body. Explaining to five-year-old Colby that Daddy was "radioactive" and couldn't hug him for a day was part of the "new normal" world I would be living in for the next six months of treatment.

Pax greeted me with another lick when I got back in the car for the drive home.

Thursday at 8:30 a.m. – CT Scan with Contrast

Have you ever had to drink a quart of barium sulfate? That's what I got to do in preparation for the CT scans on Day 3 of the testing.

Actually, CT scans are pretty basic and nothing to be afraid of. *CT* stands for "computed tomography." This test uses special x-ray equipment to obtain cross-sectional pictures of your body (Cancer.gov). Dr. Justice ordered these tests done in the pelvic and abdominal regions of my body to determine how far my cancer had spread. Together with the PET scan I had done earlier, the two tests give a complete picture of the internal organs, bones, and tissue, a picture that further helps doctors decide on a course of treatment.

The night before the test I drank a pint of barium sulfate ($BaSO_4$), which comes from the mineral barite. Barium (Ba) is #56 on the periodic table of elements chart. It's a reactive type of metal that, when combined with sulfate, becomes an ideal radio contrast agent, a medical fluid that improves the visibility of internal bodily structures in an x-ray. Because of the high atomic number of barium, the barium sulfate mixture absorbs x-rays more completely than other agents, making it ideal for showing cancer hot spots. At the time of my testing, I received another pint to drink, a white chalky fluid available in "berry flavor." Before going into the testing room, I was instructed to go to the bathroom and urinate what I could.

The CT scan test was similar to the PET scan in that I was told to lie down on a bed that traveled through the barrel of a big machine. I was strapped onto the bed and covered with a blanket for warmth, but with this test, I wasn't able to take a nap. The CT scan machine makes a whirring sound like a centrifuge as it takes pictures. I was also instructed by the technician to hold my breath at various points so that the pictures would come out nice and clear. I wasn't at all uncomfortable. I just had to hold my breath and keep my body still for several seconds at a time. The test was over in about fifteen minutes. Only the last day of testing remained.

Friday at 10:30 a.m. – Spinal Tap

"I'd rather get a spinal tap than_____ (fill in the blank)"—or so the joke goes.

I didn't know the exact purpose of a spinal tap or how the procedure was actually performed, but I already knew I didn't like it. It's sort of like disliking liver without ever trying it. You just hear enough bad things about spinal taps that you know you won't like it. I envisioned a diminutive doctor with a small, stainless steel ball-peen hammer tapping away at the base of my spine for Lord knows what reason. I remember the movie *This Is Spinal Tap* which lampooned a fictional rock band, ostensibly named for the excruciating music the band performed at eardrum-popping decibels. In truth, I knew nothing about the procedure outside of the fact that my gut told me I didn't want to have it done.

But I knew that getting an accurate diagnosis required determining exactly where the cancer cells were and weren't. Not only was I to get the dreaded spinal tap in the morning, but I was also scheduled for a bone marrow aspiration in the afternoon. Unlike the morning of the CT scan, today I was very nervous and fearful about these two procedures.

A spinal tap, also known as a lumbar puncture, is done to collect and examine the cerebrospinal fluid (CSF) that surrounds the brain and spinal cord. A needle is inserted into the spinal canal in the lower back. Fluid is drained and the samples are studied for color, blood cell counts, protein, and glucose, and the pressure of the CSF is measured as well. This procedure helps doctors determine whether symptoms are caused by infection, inflammation, or, yes, cancer (WebMD).

In spite of my apprehension, the power of prayer came to my rescue. You can just feel it! Knowing that Barbi, my family, and my church were all praying for me, I began to relax as I waited to be called. I felt very calm by the time I was called to the examining room.

After explaining the procedure, the doctor asked me to lie on my side with my knees pulled up against my chest. Curled up in the fetal position, I was then given an injection of lidocaine to numb my lower back. I experienced some mild discomfort—a brief burning sensation—before the doctor inserted a long, hollow needle into my spinal canal. The doctor then removed the center plug of the needle and fluid began to drip out. The fluid was collected in different vials for testing. The doctor also put a manometer at the end of the needle to test the fluid "pressure" just as if he were testing the oil pressure on a car.

There's really no discomfort after the initial shot, but the thought of your spinal fluid dripping out of your spinal column can be a little unsettling. So, as I did during all my tests, I just tried to focus and pray that everything would be all right, and I reminded myself that God's in charge. The whole appointment lasted thirty minutes, but the actual test took only about ten, and then I was free to go home. The procedure wasn't nearly as painful as I'd anticipated. I was told to lie down for a couple hours at home to minimize the risk of headache due to the loss of spinal fluid.

Bottom line, the spinal tap didn't live up to its villainous billing. It really was nothing to worry about.

Friday at 4:30 p.m. – Bone Marrow Aspiration

Barbi drove me down to Hoag Hospital for my last test of the week, a bone marrow aspiration. I was apprehensive about this test as well because of the less-than-comfortable bone marrow biopsy I'd had the week before. It was here at Hoag, however, that my nurse Virginia had so caringly squeezed my hand with assurance that "Everything would be okay." With that reminder, I began to relax.

The atmosphere in the doctor's office at 4:30 on a Friday

afternoon was almost festive. I was the last appointment of the day, and staff members were in a jovial mood. The Xanax Dr. J had given me to take before the examination really helped ease my nervousness. The casual atmosphere was also comforting, and it somehow made my exam—my entire situation—a little less scary.

Once on the examining table, I was asked to lie on my side. The doctor was going to remove bone marrow from my posterior iliac spine region, an area just above my right buttock. The bone marrow fluid would then undergo morphological examination to determine any irregularities in the blood cells.

The nurse gave me a numbing shot of lidocaine into the tissue next to my pelvic bone. More of a dull pressure than a sharp sting, it only hurt briefly. Once I was numb, a bone marrow aspirate needle was inserted into the numbed area and pushed into the hollow of my pelvic bone. The needle has a stylet, a thin metal probe seated inside the hollow needle. When the stylet is removed, the doctor can then affix a syringe plunger to the needle and remove the aspirate.

Unlike the spinal fluid acquired during a spinal tap, the bone marrow aspirate does not drip out on its own. It needs to be *sucked out*. As the doctor prepared to withdraw the stylet from the needle, he cautioned me with "You may feel a brief shock. Ready?" I nodded and then—WHAM! I felt a sudden, searing jolt as if my backside had been stuck into a light socket. But then, just as quickly, the pain subsided—and I experienced absolutely no lingering effects. It was literally a millisecond of pain. The electric shock I felt was my body's reaction when the doctor removed the stylet and sucked out the aspirate from my pelvic bone. To the doctor's credit, the pain was brief—and I thanked God!

One of the things you learn during your battle with cancer is that you are much stronger than you probably give yourself credit for. After the procedure was over, I was sweating, but I'd made it through—and I was relieved. In fact, with God's help, I had made it through the entire week of testing. Thanks to the prayers of my family and others (I was definitely praying too!), the professional care of dedicated nurses, doctors, and technicians, the companionship of my dog Pax, significant God-given dreams, and His truly amazing and very abundant grace, I was fortified and enabled to face the gripping fear of cancer and its companion, uncertainty. I was in capable hands—both human and divine—and I felt it.

With a yet-to-be-determined amount of chemotherapy to come and the uncertainty of all that was ahead, I could not imagine facing this alone. If you're still at odds with God over your cancer, please, please, please *humble yourself* and invite God into the situation. He wants to help you.

Learning from Job

Remember Job from the Bible? Job was a prosperous farmer living in the land of Uz. He had thousands of sheep, camels, and other livestock, a large family, and many servants—and Job lost everything. He lost his children, his position in the community, and his possessions even though he was an upright man whom God loved. Besides losing his loved ones and his reputation, Job developed sores over his whole body that were so horrible that he wanted to die.

Job was furious about his predicament. So indignant was he about the circumstances that God had allowed, Job self-righteously proclaimed:

> *"Let God weigh me in honest scales, and he will know that I am blameless."*
>
> Job 31:6

In other words, "What the heck did I do to deserve this, God?"

Maybe you can sympathize with Job. In fact, you may be terrified and/or furious at God about the road before you. After all, what did you do to deserve this?

Job continued:

> *"Oh, that I had someone to hear me!*
>
> *I sign now my defense–let the Almighty answer me; let my accuser put his indictment in writing.*
>
> *Surely, I would wear it on my shoulder, I would put it on like a crown.*
>
> *I would give him an account of my every step."*
>
> Job 31:35-37

So why does God allow us to suffer? We may not get a satisfactory answer while we're here on earth, but we need to have the courage to still trust God. If you're having doubts about God's capabilities, take a moment and listen to what God said to a self-righteous Job:

> *"Where were you when I laid the earth's foundation?...*
>
> *Who marked off its dimensions? Surely you know!*
>
> *Who stretched a measuring line across it?...*
>
> *Have you ever given orders to the morning,*
>
> *or shown the dawn its place...*
>
> *Can you bring forth the constellations in their seasons*
>
> *Or lead out the Bear with its cubs?...*
>
> *Do you send the lightning bolts on their way?"*
>
> Job 38:4-5, 12, 32, 35

Humbling words from our heavenly Father! God is simply, yet powerfully pointing out who Job isn't and who God is. Nothing—absolutely nothing—is impossible with God! His tool collection is unlimited and His power, unmatched! As these questions show, nobody thinks bigger than the Lord. Have you ever thought about any of these three issues God raised with Job? You may question a God you cannot see, but He speaks with His authority and from an eternal, all-knowing perspective.

The majesty and power of God's inquiries shook Job to the core:

"How can I reply to you?

I put my hand over my mouth."

Job 40:4

Challenge yourself to put aside your hurt, anger, and fear and to trust God with your life. He *can* save you. In my case, the Creator of all things blessed me with powerful and comforting dreams that enabled me to face my fears, trust in His strength, and rest in His peace. He also blessed me with doctors, clinicians, technology, testing, and medicines to diagnose my cancer and treat it.

But what about a cure? you may ask. *Will God cure me?*

You can debate the answer to this question however you like, but from my perspective, that really isn't the main issue. The main issue is *Will you crumble under your fear of cancer, will you tough it out on your own, or will you turn to the One who created you and choose to trust in Him?*

It's puzzling to me—and it can be tragic—that people try to do life without God, yet I understand it because I do the same thing! Sometimes, for instance, I let myself think that God is either distant or uninterested in my situation. I use this rationale to justify making decisions without asking God for His input or guidance. Other times I get too comfortable with the peace and success that God has blessed me with. Then I start to believe that I myself am the reason for my success and that I can handle life on my own. What an utterly misguided and false belief!

My cancer, however, reminded me that not only am I unable to manage the circumstances and situations in my life, but I am also completely incapable of controlling whatever is going on inside my own body. Cancer reminded me of how truly weak I am, yet it gave me opportunity after opportunity to see how truly strong and good God is. What a blessing our Lord is in times of trouble! He faithfully responds whenever we call on Him!

Quite simply, choosing to accept the reality of God's strength, power, and love—choosing to trust in His sovereignty over your life and your disease—is the first serious step a person diagnosed with cancer or any life-threatening illness can take toward winning the battle.

Chapter 7

"Have a *Little* Faith"

WHEN MY TEST RESULTS WERE IN, DR. JUSTICE SHARED THEM with his colleagues at the Norris Comprehensive Cancer Center. After a thorough review of the scans, tests, and slides, the experts confirmed what the Hoag doctors had concluded: I had PTCL-NOS. More specifically, I had Non-Hodgkin's Peripheral T-cell Lymphoma, Intermediate Grade, NOS (Not Otherwise Specified). The cancer—stage 4—was present on my right seventh rib and throughout my lymph nodes in my underarms, neck, and chest. My right underarm—the one that had been sore and diagnosed initially as a "blocked sweat gland"—was actually a cancerous lymph node.

According to an article on T-cell lymphoma published in PubMed.gov, the median age for PTCL-NOS is fifty-five to sixty years old, and it occurs mostly in males. When the study was published in August 2010, the five-year survival rate was approximately 25%. Not the best odds, but truthfully, as long as there was a cure rate of any kind, I didn't care what the odds were. I had made a decision in Dr. Collins' office that even if there were only a 1% cure rate, I was going to be in that 1%.

That declaration was a defining moment in my life. My wife and my young sons needed me, and I was terrified of leaving them alone. I was more terrified of leaving them alone than I was of dying. Was I going to run from cancer in fear, or was I going to stand up to it in faith? For my family's sake, I was going to stand up to cancer and fight—but at the same time, I was terrified. I was afraid of the cancer, but I knew that God wasn't. My cancer may have been bigger than I was, but it was not bigger than God—and never in all my life had I believed anything as strongly as I believed that.

With the diagnosis confirmed, I was to begin CHOP chemotherapy immediately, every three weeks, for six months. In light of my relative health, Dr. J would maximize the dosages to give me the best chance of killing off my cancer permanently. "We don't want this coming back," reasoned Dr. J.

CHOP—one of the most common chemotherapy regimens for treating Non-Hodgkin's lymphoma—involves four drugs: Cytoxan, Hydroxydoxorubicin, Oncovin, and Prednisone. My chemotherapy would add the drug Rituxan, so technically my regimen was CHOP+R. (Each of these drugs has different brand names. In my case, for instance, I received Vincristine, which was equivalent to Oncovin.)

I knew that the side effects of chemo were bad. I had heard of people vomiting nonstop, losing their hair, feeling fatigued, losing muscle mass, and basically feeling like crap as they wasted away due to the drugs. Sterility was another side effect.... This treatment wasn't like being sick for a week or two and then feeling better. I was faced with losing my strength, losing my health, and, most importantly, losing my life and, with it, my family.

I believed I would survive, but how would I be able to endure the six months of hell that stretched before me? I wanted to run home, bury my head under the covers, and be told everything would be all right in the morning. How would I be able to face, much less conquer, the challenges that lay ahead?

Taking Trust to a New Level

I was overwhelmed when I considered all that was before me. One moment I would feel the strength of God and be absolutely confident in His ability to heal me, but the next I would remember that there are no guarantees and that this is damn scary stuff. Clearly, I would not be able to fight this battle alone, and I would really need to lean on God with more than just words and pronouncements. I would, literally, need to trust Him with my life.

I thought about the time Jesus' disciples were in a small boat on the Sea of Galilee. Jesus had sent them ahead to the other side so He could have time by Himself to pray. Later that night a wind came up, and the disciples' boat was being tossed about by the waves. In the distance, they saw what looked like a ghost walking across the water. They were terrified.

"It's a ghost," they said, and cried out in fear. But Jesus immediately said to them: "Take courage! It is I. Don't be afraid."

"Lord, if it's you," Peter replied, "tell me to come to you on the water."

"Come," he said.

Then Peter got down out of the boat, walked on the water and came toward Jesus. But when he saw the wind, he was afraid and, beginning to sink, cried out, "Lord, save me!"

Immediately Jesus reached out his hand and caught him. "You of little faith," he said, "why did you doubt?"

Matthew 14:26-31

Peter doubted for the same reason I doubted: because he was human and he was afraid! Peter briefly experienced a spiritual law that defied gravity—and he walked on water! When he realized what he was doing, though, his finite mind took over, and he began to sink. Peter doubted just as we all do when we're attempting something we haven't done before.

For me, another picture of fear comes to mind…. Every year my mom and dad rent a cabin at Donner Lake. It's a terrific old cabin, large enough to house several families. Situated on the northeast end of the lake, it has a small pier in a protected cove where we dock a couple boats and swim and play. Although my mom and dad have been divorced for over thirty years now, everyone still goes up to the cabin—new spouses, stepchildren, everyone—to enjoy the beautiful surroundings and the fun of being with family.

For the kids—and for the young at heart—the most prized recreational opportunity is running the length of the pier and jumping off the end. Depending on how much water was let out of the lake that year, the drop ranges between three and five feet. The water is a deep forest green but clear enough that you can see the sandy lake bottom as you stand on the pier.

When my son Colby was four years old, he was ready to take part in this family tradition. His brothers and cousins and assorted relatives were all running the length of the pier and jumping into the refreshing (some say "ice cold") water. Then they swam around the dock, climbed out of the water, and sprinted down the pier for another jump in the lake. Colby had a problem, though: he couldn't bring himself to jump. He was paralyzed with fear.

Even though Colby saw his brothers and cousins running and jumping and laughing and totally surviving their leaps into the lake, he could not bring himself to leave the safety of the pier and jump in. If you really got to the heart of matter, Colby could not bring himself to believe that he would survive. Despite encouragement from everyone there, Colby stood frozen like a Popsicle. My son was afraid to make the leap just as Peter was, just as I was, and—more than likely—just as you are in your particular battle. Yet how wonderfully God provides us with the gift of helping hands. We never need to face our challenges alone.

And in those challenging circumstances, sometimes God catches us, but sometimes He outright pushes us. When Peter realized he was sinking in the Sea of Galilee and cried out to Jesus, the Lord reached out His hand and caught him. Peter survived.

In Colby's case, however, he needed a push, and God determined that his father would administer the push! I held Colby's hand and helped him. Okay, I pushed him. He survived. And once Colby discovered he could survive the leap off the pier, he was like a Tasmanian devil, running and jumping and splashing and whirring about in utter chaotic delight, no longer paralyzed by a debilitating fear.

Figuratively speaking, how was I going to survive my jump from the pier? How will you survive yours?

"Have a *Little* Faith"

As I was considering these things, I went for a walk. I needed to talk to Jesus. For me, talking to Jesus is the same as talking to God. I actually walked the boys to school first, which was just a short five-minute stroll down the street and across the boulevard that borders our development to the north. After I saw the boys off to their classrooms, I continued walking around the neighborhood. I find that when I go for a jog or a walk, when I can get away from everything, my prayer dialogue with Jesus is the richest. I simply talk to Him, either silently or aloud, as if He were walking right next to me. As I mentioned earlier, I was feeling shaky, overwhelmed by all that was before me, so I started talking to Jesus about those concerns—and I got an immediate reply that stopped me in my tracks: "Rob, have a *little* faith."

What's that? Have a little faith?

"Rob, have a *little* faith," I heard Jesus say again. I didn't hear an audible voice, but in my mind's eye—or ear, rather—those were exactly the Lord's words: "Rob, have a *little* faith." I heard this as meaning "Come on, Rob. I'm Jesus. I can walk on water and raise the dead. Have a *little* faith in Me."

I was taken aback by the way I heard Jesus' words, as if curing my cancer and walking me through the chemo journey were no big deal for Him, as if I were asking the Lord to do a menial task: "Have a *little* faith." Jesus caught me completely and wonderfully off guard. Of course Jesus can cure my cancer. He's God!

"OK," I said, playing along. "OK, Jesus, I can have a *little* faith. I can't have this big and perfect faith, like Abraham or Moses or the apostle Paul, but a *little* faith I can have." Then I remembered the parable about the mustard seed:

"Though it is the smallest of all seeds, yet when it grows, it is the largest of garden plants and becomes a tree so that the birds come and perch in its branches."

Jesus in Matthew 12:32

Faith like a mustard seed. Not big and perfect faith, but a little *faith—that seems very doable.... I can do that!*

Jesus taught that small beginnings can yield great results, and my having a *little* faith would be that small beginning for me. I wanted to believe that Jesus was telling me He would heal me, but I still had to think through all this and get my mind around what it all meant. *Was Jesus actually saying He would heal me? Or was He talking about something else? What was Jesus trying to tell me?* To be honest, I was fearful and unsure, but at the same time it felt right to trust Jesus to "have a *little* faith," so I decided to risk it.

OK, Lord, I said to Him more seriously this time. *I can have a* little *faith.*

Once I got to this point—once I decided to trust the Lord just enough to accept His invitation to have a *little* faith—I was blessed with two more thoughts from Him: *Have a plan* and *Follow the plan.* I no longer felt overwhelmed. Jesus had just given me a three-step plan:

1. Have a *little* faith.

2. Have a plan.

3. Follow the plan.

By God's grace, the second and third steps were already in place: I had gotten the best doctor I could, and I was following his plan. I had no doubt that God had guided me to Dr. J. And just as there had been nothing random about my connecting with Dr. J, there would be nothing random about this skilled doctor's course of action.

Notice how Jesus changed my focus from "Woe is me! How am I going to do this?" to "Have a *little* faith." I was looking for sympathy for my cause; Jesus was looking for faith in His. I wanted comfort; Jesus wanted action. I shared a concern: "I'm afraid! Help me!" Jesus shared a challenge: "Have a *little* faith and trust Me." At this point I started to understand—because I was living it—that God does not always give us what we want, but He gives us what we need. God simply knows what's best for us.

Nailing Step #1

I realized I had to take on more responsibility regarding the first step of this three-step plan. The "have a *little* faith" component required me to have a more positive mindset and to do things that would fuel that healthier, more helpful mindset. So I made the decision—and I made the commitment to myself—that I would be stronger, mentally as well as physically, at the end of chemo than I was at the start. I was not going to waste away and complain about all the chemo "destroying" my body. It was clear to me that since Jesus was willing to do His part in my battle against cancer, I needed to be willing to do my part. In other words, I came to the conclusion that I could not expect the Lord to heal me if I had a negative, faithless attitude.

I also decided that I would make this change in attitude evident on two fronts. First, I would exercise daily: I would do pushups, play tennis or golf, jog, walk, do anything I could to remain physically fit. Second, I would not—as an act of trust that the Lord would heal me—give further voice to my fears or belabor my doubts. Neither would I discuss the "realistic" outcomes of treatment suggested by statistics. I didn't care what the statistics were. I didn't care what the effects of chemotherapy were. I didn't care what "the world" thought about cancer or about how I should manage it. I cared about only one thing: *believing that I was curable and doing things that demonstrated that belief.*

Life-Giving Prayer

At this point I want to say something about prayer. First, prayer is basically having an open conversation with God. Of course, going to church is a good thing, but you don't need to go to church on Sunday to be with God or pray to Him. You can be with God any day of the week, anytime, anywhere. Even now our omniscient Lord is looking forward to hearing from you. God loves you, He loves listening to you, He loves talking to you, and He loves blessing you.

> *"Ask and it will be given to you; seek and you will find; knock and the door will be opened to you."*
>
> Jesus in Luke 11:9

Why should we be surprised that, when we ask God for something, when we seek His counsel, when we knock on His door for help, He will respond?

"But," you may be screaming this inside, "God doesn't heal everyone. It's not that easy! People die! And since God doesn't heal everyone, what am I having faith in?"

You may know some God-fearing friends or relatives who

believed in the Lord, who trusted Him
who were not healed. "What about the
If this is your case, I'm very sorry for yo

I asked God the same question a
matter. The minister of my church did

Dr. John Huffman, then senior pastor at
Presbyterian in Newport Beach, California, lost his beautiful
daughter Suzanne to cancer when she was nineteen. She
was a sophomore at Princeton University when she was
diagnosed with a relatively minor cancer, one that had a 98%
cure rate. Suzanne had grown up in the Christian faith and
was loved by many. She had the prayers of our five-thousand-
member congregation behind her. Suzanne was a thoughtful,
generous person who loved the Lord. No doubt she invoked
all the powerful Scriptures she knew to bolster her faith as she
prayed to God for healing. And she died.

I remember John's wife, Anne, on stage at church speaking
openly about how angry she was at God for taking her
daughter from her. Loved ones do die, and some are taken
from us far too early. I don't have a good answer as to why
God allows some people to die much too soon and others to
enjoy a long, vibrant life. I don't have a good answer as to
why God allows some people to live longer than others. I also
don't have a good answer as to why He allows the profound
suffering experienced by parents who bury their children. One
thing I know for sure, though, is that God doesn't determine
whether He will heal a person on the basis of that person
being good or bad. Plenty of "good" people die young, and
plenty of "bad" people die old. But I do know that God calls

ɔ have faith in Him, to trust in the goodness of His
ıd to leave the outcome in His hands.

My good friend Laura passed away from ovarian cancer
after a five-year battle and more than 200 rounds of chemo.
I was in seventh grade when Laura was my first girlfriend
and the first girl I kissed. When Laura found out after her
Herculean battle that she would be dying soon, she heroically
began planning her funeral and asked me to speak. Laura had
come to peace with God's plan even though it meant leaving
behind her husband of twenty-five years and their beloved
son Bryan, who was twenty years old. How did Laura come
to a place of trusting God even when that place meant her life
on earth would end? Laura could have asked, "What good
is faith?" and rejected God for not answering her prayer to
beat cancer, but Laura believed that there was more life to
come! Look at the Scripture passage she asked me to read at
her funeral:

> *"So we do not lose heart. Though our outer self
> is wasting away, our inner self is renewed day
> by day. For this light momentary affliction is
> preparing for us an eternal weight of glory beyond
> all comparison, as we look not to the things that
> are seen but to the things that are unseen. For the
> things that are seen are transient, but the things
> that are unseen are eternal."*
>
> 2 Corinthian 4:16-18 ESV

This is not the belief of someone beaten by cancer! This statement reflects the belief of one who has conquered cancer. Oh, cancer may have won a round, but it never beat Laura! A warrior from the start, Laura used cancer to show her loved ones on earth how to live by faith. Her faith also clearly communicated her confidence that this life is not all there is to life!

> *"Do not let your hearts be troubled. Trust in God; trust also in me. In my Father's house are many rooms; if it were not so, I would have told you. I am going there to prepare a place for you. And if I go and prepare a place for you, I will come back and take you to be with me that you also may be where I am."*
>
> Jesus in John 14:1-3

Jesus loves you, and He wants to fight for your life just as He wants to fight for mine. I needed to make peace with the Lord that I would trust Him no matter what happened. As I said in the examination room in Dr. Collins' office that first day, "If it's my time to go, then it's my time to go, but God isn't afraid of cancer—and I'm not going to run in fear of it either." Despite the odds, despite the uncertainties, despite the stresses of having a life-threatening disease, I needed to consider all the possible consequences and make a solid decision about how I would approach this battle. I didn't want to fight this battle alone. I decided to trust God. I decided to trust Jesus and have faith that He and Father God—my

Creator and the Great Physician—would heal me. Having faith is not easy. But if we only had faith when the situation has a known outcome that we approve of, it wouldn't really be faith, would it?

"We live by faith, not by sight."

2 Corinthians 5:7

The Blessing of Barbi

"You're going to survive," Barbi said.

We were still in the early stage of our cancer fight, and we'd just gotten into bed. Barbi said it again: "You're going to survive this cancer." Then she added, "I had a premonition."

I looked right at my wife and felt a variety of emotions. I was thankful for her reassurance, comforted by her confident belief, and—truth be told—probably a bit skeptical. My eyes warily asked, "Are you sure?"

"I just know," Barbi continued. "I heard a voice that said, 'Rob's going to make it this time.'"

WOW!

I love my wife!

I love Barbi's strength and her faith. Although she will tell you otherwise, she is much, much stronger than I am, and I was deeply comforted by her belief that I would survive this cancer. With Barbi's steadfast belief that I was going to beat this cancer, I relaxed a little more, I believed a little more, and my faith in God grew a little more. I was greatly encouraged by Barbi's bold declaration that I was going to survive. Oh, Barbi... Oh, faith. ... Oh, God!

> *"May the God of hope fill you with all joy and peace in believing, so that by the power of the Holy Spirit you may abound in hope."*
>
> Romans 15:13 ESV

These are deep waters....-

Barbi had a premonition and heard a voice say, "Rob's going to make it this time" Barbi won't claim it was the voice of God. How could she? But it was a voice of comfort, and it was a convincing voice. It may not have been the Lord's voice, but who else could have initiated it? I've heard the Lord speak to me in my mind. As I've shared, I heard Jesus chide me to "Have a *little* faith," but I've never heard Him speak to me *audibly.*

But there it was: Barbi heard a voice telling her I would survive this cancer. So was this a voice from God—or wasn't it? Was I going to survive this cancer—or wasn't I? Would I believe in what Barbi shared with me—or wouldn't I?

> *"You of little faith, why are you so afraid?"*
>
> Jesus in Matthew 8:26

Afraid to Trust God

How hard it can be to trust God, to believe His promises, to rest in His faithfulness. Yet rather than hide what I was thinking from God (which is impossible to do anyway), I just spoke to Him honestly about my fears. I didn't hold back:

Lord, I'm afraid of dying. I'm afraid of not being strong enough. In fact, I'm totally afraid that I'll be weak and crumble. I'm afraid that I may be leaving my wife alone and financially strapped. I'm afraid of not being there for my boys when they're sad and lonely and need their father. I'm afraid of failing my family. I'm afraid of missing out on all that lies ahead for my sons. I'm afraid of losing their love and Barbi's love. I'm afraid the plan You have for my life is to take me early for some reason that will be explained in time to come. But in the present time, Your plan will rip my life and my family's lives apart in pain and agony. I'm afraid to trust You, Lord...

Some of you may be uncomfortable with this approach, as if by disclosing your fears you give God ammunition to really hurt you. But God tells us—God *commands* us—to do this:

"Cast all your anxiety on him because he cares for you."

1 Peter 5:7

To be close with God, we need to be honest with Him, and I am a witness to the truth that He can handle our honesty, our raw pain, our unfiltered rage, whatever it is we're feeling and thinking.

The Crucible of Cancer

Shortly after I was diagnosed with cancer, Barbi threw the most magical surprise birthday party to celebrate my turning forty. Returning home from work, I saw the whole street lined with cars and wondered, *Who is having such a big party?* Then I noticed my brother-in-law's car with his distinctive license plate "MR TT," and I got a lump in my throat. I knew what was coming.

When I opened the front door, I was greeted with a shout of "Surprise!" by family members and my closest friends, and, in tears, I just buried my head as I hugged Barbi. My boys, each dressed in white polo shirts, ran up to give me a hug. The party's preppy theme meant everyone assembled had donned polo shirts, madras shorts, seersucker, button-downs, Top-Siders, pink and green, Ray-Ban sunglasses—all the fun stuff from the early '80s when I was in college and the style was popular. Barbi likes to remind me that when I walked in the front door to the party, I was wearing a pink polo shirt, proof positive that my fashion sense hadn't much progressed since college!

It was the most special party I have ever attended, and we were all in good spirits. Barbi had arranged for our church pianist to play for the evening. We had passed hors d'oeuvres and a bartender serving themed drinks like Rob's Razzleberry Pinktini. Our dear family friend Mary Richardson baked 200 alligator-shaped cookies, decorating each of them with preppy green sweaters! Our friend Larry Crandall took photos of the party, some of which are included in this book. My favorite is one Larry snapped of Barbi and me looking into each other's eyes, full of love. I adore my beautiful Barbi.

After visiting with friends and relatives (some of whom I hadn't seen in years) and enjoying the food, the music and the atmosphere, we all went and stood in front of the house for a group photo. With everyone assembled, I had an opportunity to thank them for celebrating my birthday with me. And as I was thanking everyone for coming and for their support, I was filled with God-given peace and comfort. I told them that I believed God was going to heal me. I could see everyone's eyes welling up with tears as they saw this young father of three boys, stricken with life-threatening cancer, completely bald and vulnerable. And yet here I was comforting everyone else: "I believe God is going to heal me. But if He doesn't, that's OK. Either way, my family and I know that God loves us. But I do believe He will heal me."

When I put my faith in Jesus, I had given up a claim on my life. Afterward, I found comfort in the Scripture:

> *"For whoever wants to save their life will lose it, but whoever loses their life for me will find it."*
>
> Jesus in Matthew 16.25

Maybe coming to this point looks to some people like giving up and giving in, but quite the opposite is true. The choice to surrender one's life—one's self—to Jesus is a conscious step necessary for dropping a false belief ("I am sovereign") and for claiming a truth ("God is sovereign").

I need Jesus. You need Jesus. Surrender yourself to Him. Submit your own plans for your life to Him. And be saved.

"For God so loved the world that he gave his one and only Son, that whoever believes in him shall not perish but have eternal life."

Jesus in John 3:16

I chose to trust that the almighty Creator of the universe had not only the *power* to save me, but also the *desire* to save me. So I chose to have faith in Him; I chose to trust Him. And with that decision to trust God, I received exactly what the Lord promises in Scripture:

"Do not be anxious about anything, but in every situation, by prayer and petition, with thanksgiving, present your requests to God. And the peace of God, which transcends all understanding, will guard your hearts and your minds in Christ Jesus."

Philippians 4:6-7

So I slept well. I dreamt well. I experienced God's peace and His comfort. I wasn't anxious. I was strong and steadfast. I was confident. I was trusting and grateful. I was free to die—and that gave me the freedom to truly live. This is a challenging truth, but *I honestly became my best self in this crucible of cancer because of what God did for me.* I received a peace that transcended all understanding, and Jesus protected my heart and mind just as Scripture promises.

I would need this newfound strength and peace in the Lord because chemotherapy was about to begin.

Chapter 8

Chemo: Embrace It!

Chemotherapy.

We all have preconceived notions about chemo. We either know someone who has gone through it or is going through it, or we've heard stories about people who have gone through it. Perhaps you've gone through chemo, are going through it now, or are about to go through it. One way or another, we are all connected to someone's experience of chemotherapy, and we've all formulated some thoughts about what that experience is like.

At the time of my first appointment, I didn't know what each of the drugs was or any of the side effects. What I did know was that I needed this treatment to survive, so in the scheme of things, the side effects were really irrelevant. That's not to say that I wasn't concerned about the side effects. I'm just saying that I was not going to let my fear of any side effects keep me from having a positive attitude about the treatment and its life-saving benefits.

Karen Koeller and Barbi joined me for my first visit to Dr. J's office for chemo. What a blessing it was to have them there! I would highly recommend that, if at all possible, you take a family member or friend to your chemo appointments. God gives us the blessing of companionship so that we don't need to face our trials alone. For some people, arranging to have some company may require the humbling admission that you are scared and could use some comfort. Let me offer the reassurance that it is very freeing to admit our needs and to give others a chance to meet them. Having Barbi and Karen with me helped keep me from going inward to a place of doubt. Having them there helped me relax and feel more confident, more at peace.

Yet—and it sounds silly—I've always wanted to perform well in front of others. From my first swim team race when I came in fourth place, received a green ribbon, and got all the accolades from my mom and dad about what a great athlete I was, I've always sought people's approval through my athletic accomplishments, and their approval felt good.

I played baseball, basketball, and football in junior high; I was on the swim team from ages seven to fifteen and on the water polo and tennis teams in high school; and I rowed crew for a year at USC. I like people cheering for me. Even today, if someone is watching me play a game of tennis, I'll play harder. It's embarrassing to admit this, but like a child seeking his parents' approval, I still want others to think I'm special. Don't we all?

So, as I waited with Barbi and Karen, I was anxious about my first chemo, but I wanted to win the game by being courageous. I wanted to be strong for Barbi, and I didn't want our friend Karen to think I was weak. I wanted approval, and I wanted Barbi to be proud of me. And of course I wanted to live: I wanted to survive.

All In!

I began preparing my mind to win this battle by making these key choices: *Trust in God. Trust in the treatment. Trust in the doctors. Trust in myself. Nurture that desire to win.* I wanted to not merely beat this cancer. I wanted to crush it. I wanted to pulverize it. I wanted to destroy the cancer inside me—and I wanted to be physically stronger at the end of my chemotherapy than I was at the beginning.

To further strengthen myself for the battle, I associated the cancer with Satan, a dark and malicious invader who wanted to destroy me and leave my boys fatherless. I personified the cancer and would call it out: "F… you, Satan! You're *not* stronger than God! In Jesus' name, leave me!" No cancer is stronger than God, and I wanted to do my share of "having a *little* faith" as Jesus had encouraged me to have. For this battle, I was all in.

Being all in. How many times in your life have you truly been *all* in? How many times have you found everything you know and everyone you love on the line and you were willing to do whatever it took to overcome your adversary? One blessing of cancer is that it's a crucible, and as a crucible, it can purify your thoughts. Cancer clarifies what is actually important and what really matters in your life. Cancer helped me realize to a new degree that I desperately wanted to live and that I desperately wanted to be with my family. Everything else was trivial. Being focused on this outcome I so passionately wanted gave me incredible purpose, motivation, and strength. For the first time in my life, I knew with absolute certainty what I wanted, and it was life with Barbi and my boys.

The Waiting Room

Back in Dr. J's office, about a half dozen others waited to be called for their appointments, some for doctor's visits and others for chemotherapy. The spirit of the reception area was a mixture of concern, acceptance, and hope. I noticed the uneasiness and anxiety of new patients and the odd type of acceptance and peace of veteran patients. As Karen, Barbi, and I waited in the reception area, warmly furnished with comfortable chairs and couches, we asked God to give me comfort and strength and to make my treatments effective.

Shortly after our prayer, a gentleman came into the reception area holding in his hand a slip of paper from the doctor. Pausing in the middle of the room, he looked at that paper and exclaimed, "Thank God! Six months of chemo, and it's all gone! My wife's cancer is in full remission!" Everyone in the room clapped for him, and he left crying tears of joy.

I was greatly encouraged by this man's announcement. His wife's experience gave me hope: people in this very room were being cured of cancer. Perhaps it was a coincidence that this man walked through the waiting room with such great news while we were sitting there awaiting my first treatment, but perhaps not. I do know, however, that the more I pray, the more I trust in God, and the more I call on Him to help me, the more blessings "coincidentally" occur in my life.

A nurse appeared and called me in for my first treatment. I got up from my chair with increasing confidence in my God.

Weighing In

Every doctor visit and chemo session began with getting weighed. Apart from the fact that I had stage 4 lymphoma, I was in decent shape at 6'0" and 180 pounds. Keeping that weight on would be very important to my treatment and cure. Yet—as I soon learned—chemo diminished my appetite, and food didn't taste as good. (Now don't get excited and think of using chemo as a chance to lose weight. Your doctor will probably caution you not to do so.)

According to "Expert Voices at the American Cancer Society" (cancer.org), weight loss during chemo can reduce both your energy and the much-needed nutrients your body stores. Because chemo kills off both bad cells and good ones, your body has to work harder to repair the tissue damage caused by chemo. If you don't have sufficient weight, the energy and proteins needed to repair chemo-damaged tissue will be taken from your lean body muscle, further decreasing your stamina. And you need your stamina as the cancer and the chemo war against each other in the battleground of your body. "I don't care if you need to eat McDonald's hamburgers and milkshakes to keep the weight on," Dr. Justice had told me earlier. "Do it."

Meet Cindy

As we walked back to the chemo ward, the doctor's office was a beehive of activity. Dr. Justice was busy on the phone, but he made a point to stop me, give me a hug, and welcome me. "I want to make sure you come see me after your visit today," he said as if I were the only one in the room. Dr. J had the incredible gift of making each one of his patients feel important.

The chemo ward itself is a light- and life-filled room of windows, La-Z-Boy recliners, and people of varying ages, ethnicities, and stages of cancer. The nurses were moving about as if they were in a MASH unit, inserting IVs, checking saline bags, delivering blankets, helping patients to the restroom, infusing drugs, passing out water and Ensure bottles (to help patients maintain their weight), and adjusting pillows, TV channels, and volume. But what the oncology nurses—and patients—took the most delight in delivering was… banter. The nurses were incredibly sensitive about being sure we patients were comfortable, and they were delivering top-notch professional treatment. But in the chemo ward, if anyone had any hair left, this is where they would let it down! The banter was a way of humorously dealing with a very harsh reality.

Cancer is serious business, but cutting the tension that everyone felt was a back-and-forth banter between the patients and the nurses. The banter also served the more poignant role of preventing anyone from getting sucked into the debilitating black hole of self-pity. It's tough to feel sorry for yourself when everyone else is in the same boat, when everyone's life is at stake. The message was "Get a grip and fight like the rest of us!" The chemo room truly is one of the most life-affirming environments I've ever been in.

The lead nurse's name was Cindy. She was all of five feet tall and 100 pounds, but she was feisty. "Hey, Cindy! Could you turn the channel? I can't stand *AM Los Angeles*," someone would bellow.

"Change it yourself!" Cindy would bark in return. "I'm not changing it. That's my favorite show." Various people would snicker, and soon others would join in to get her going.

"Hey, Cindy! My bag's empty. What are you trying to do? Kill me?"

"Hold your horses, Charles! You're not dead yet!" she'd fire back.

As I was paying attention to the rapid-fire banter going on in the room, I began to relax and settle into my La-Z-Boy recliner. Barbi and Karen sat in chairs next to me, and their presence was very reassuring. I was definitely ready to get things underway.

Cindy came up and introduced herself. Like Dr. J, Cindy made me feel like the most special person in the room. Somehow she could take care of me even as, in her tough Italian way, she was responding to patient requests and fending off verbal barbs. Whenever she had a good comeback ("What am I, your mother?"), she'd wink and smile at me as if I were in on the joke. I liked Cindy instantly. Clearly, she didn't want her patients to feel sorry for themselves. Instead, she wanted each one of us to fight and to believe in our ability to survive—and she was just the person to help make that happen. Patients absolutely loved Cindy because, first, she wouldn't take any guff and, second, she always gave 110%. It was very clear that Cindy genuinely wanted the best for each one of us.

As tough as Cindy was, she knew there were people in her care who would not survive long. She knew which people were suffering the way no one should ever have to suffer. She saw her patients wince with pain as she poked around to find a vein that had closed. The work she did had to take a tremendous emotional toll on her each and every day. Her tough talk was a defense mechanism. We all knew it, and we loved her for it. I imagine Cindy was like the Holly Hunter character in the 1987 movie *Broadcast News* who went home each night and cried herself to sleep over the stresses of the day. We were in this place to get healed, and Cindy was going to hold us accountable to that. She would save her tears for later, when she was away from her patients. What a gift Cindy was to Dr. J's chemo patients.

The Nuts and Bolts of Chemo

Cindy went over my CHOP+R treatment—Cytoxan, Hydroxydoxorubicin (Adriamycin), Oncovin (Vincristine), Prednisone, and Rituxin. During my six months of chemo, my routine was full chemo and Rituxin every three weeks, followed by a Rituxin-only treatment every other week.

"After you go into remission, if anything comes back, we zap it with Rituxin, and you're good to go," Cindy said encouragingly. In Cindy's description of the treatment, it was a foregone conclusion that we'd beat this cancer into submission and that, if something came back, a dose of Rituxin would take care of it. It remained to be seen how difficult the treatment would be, but I believed Cindy and took comfort in her words.

I was first given an IV with a saline drip bag. Cindy would need to find a vein in my right or left arm, and she selected a vein on the back of my left hand. She was pleased that I had "good veins." (Sometimes with older patients, nurses can have a hard time finding a vein to insert the IV needle into—and if they do, the insertion can be painful. If this is your situation or if you will be getting more frequent chemos, you may be given a port-a-cath. This surgically-installed catheter allows nurses to administer chemo and to draw blood without poking the veins in your arms or hands.)

In my case, Cindy gave me a small poke and got the needle in my vein effortlessly. I barely felt it. "We use baby needles," Cindy winked. "They're smaller in diameter so you don't feel it as much." Cindy next taped down the IV so it wouldn't dislodge if I accidentally knocked into it. So far, so good!

The first drug I received was Cytoxin, and a bag of it was hung next to my saline bag. The tubes have valves that open and close, so the nurse can stop the flow of saline and begin the flow of Cytoxin. The administration of Cytoxin would take about thirty minutes or so. I said a prayer as I watched the clear fluid drip... drip... drip... from the bag... down the tube... through the IV that was inserted in my left hand... and into my veins. Glad that there was no pain during this process, I began to relax a bit more. With Barbi and Karen there in the room with me, I felt I needed to be good company and keep up with the conversation. Thankfully, they both recognized what I was trying to do and gave me permission to just relax and rest. "You don't need to entertain us," Barbi said reassuringly.

When my bag was empty, the Cytoxin was closed and the saline valve reopened. I made sure to advise Cindy when the Cytoxin tube was empty because I was fearful of air being sucked into my veins. Although Cindy assured me that couldn't happen, it was an anxiety I nevertheless carried throughout my chemo.

The next medicine was the aptly named Adriamycin push. The Adriamycin comes in a big syringe, about 1 ½" in diameter and 8" long. The oncology nurse inserts the needle into the saline tube and pushes the Adriamycin into the IV. Remember the gelatinous red-pink hair styling gel Dippity Do with what looked like clear air bubbles interspersed throughout it? That's what the Adriamycin looks like, but it was not at all Dippity Do gentle. Imagine a high-octane, industrial-grade solvent, something that strips varnish in a single swipe, and you'll have a sense of the power of Adriamycin. Making friends with Adriamycin was like making friends with the schoolyard bully who could destroy enemies with a mere glance. I made quick friends with the bad-ass Adriamycin.

After a half hour or so of Adriamycin, I was to get a push of Vincristine, but first I had to go to the bathroom. Because you are taking in several liters of saline along with the chemo meds, you are regularly going to the bathroom to eliminate the fluids. I loved this, especially after the Adriamycin push.

First of all—and maybe it's different for guys than girls—the relief of taking a good pee is really satisfying. And even more satisfying was seeing the red-tinged hue of my urine, giving visual evidence that the Adriamycin was kicking ass and bloodying up the opponent as it worked its way through my system. I envisioned teams of cancer cells being caught up in that Adriamycin stream and then shot out —and then flushed down the toilet for good. "F-you, cancer!"

Vincristine was the last medicine Cindy would push into my IV. (Prednisone came in a pill form. More on that in a minute.) This drug interferes with the growth of cancer cells and slows their spread in the body. An anti-neoplastic drug, Vincristine hates neoplastic cancer cells and kills them. Able to relax a bit knowing this was the final infusion of the day, I actually drifted off to sleep. The comfortable La-Z-Boy recliner, the warm blanket, my wife Barbi by my side, and the comfort of knowing that I was in God's hands lulled me into a restful sleep.

Yes, restful. Sleeping restfully in a cancer treatment room sounds so contrary to what I expected. After all, having this peace, this confidence, is not my natural bent. I would characterize myself as a cautious optimist at best—and a self-flagellating doubter at worst. For me to feel confident that I could beat cancer, confident that I could beat chemo by being stronger than its side effects, was the work of the Lord and completely His gracious provision. I trusted God, and He answered my prayer. Despite fear and doubt and the odds against my survival screaming at me, I *chose* to place my trust in Jesus and *believe*.

"I can do all things through Christ who strengthens me."

Philippians 4:13 NKJV

The Value of a Picture

We've all heard it said that a picture is worth a thousand words. This is true in the treatment of cancer: visualization would prove very important in my battle.

So, I visualized cancer being like sand caked on my seventh rib. I pictured my rib being a pillar of marble, strong and nonporous. I visualized the chemo as water coming out of a hose and washing away the cancerous sand immediately upon contact. Sometimes I lost the image of my rib as a marble pillar, and instead I saw the cancerous sand lodge into a fissure in my rib. So, then I visualized a surgeon cutting into my rib and carving out the cancer. I also visualized squeezing the cancer out from my rib like a pustule and then slicing off the roots. Each time the cancer wanted to stick to my rib or reattach itself, I visualized a fire hose blasting water at it, a knife slicing it, fire burning it, anything that destroyed the cancer—and seeing washed it from my body. I then pictured the cancer cells, like soapy water dirty after a shower, being rinsed down the drain for good.

The P in CHOP+R

I took the prednisone in pill form at home. My regimen started with five 20-mg pills, and I reduced the number of pills one pill per day for five days. Originally developed as an anti-inflammatory alternative to cortisone, Prednisone was used by people suffering from rheumatoid arthritis. It was later discovered that Prednisone had several beneficial side effects. Prednisone can stimulate appetite, help you keep weight on, and build muscle during your chemo. Prednisone also causes cancer cells to commit suicide:

> **Prednisone is a type of steroid drug known as a glucocorticosteroid. It is a man-made version of a natural hormone produced by the adrenal glands. Glucocorticosteroids have a wide range of actions on many parts of the body. The ways in which they cause these many different effects aren't exactly clear.**
>
> **The main effects of prednisone and steroids like it seem to be due to their anti-inflammatory properties and their ability to alter immune system responses. For example, prednisone helps prevent white blood cells from traveling to areas of the body where they might add to swelling problems (such as around tumors). It also seems to help with the treatment of certain blood cancers (such as leukemia) by causing some cancerous white blood cells to commit suicide. (American Cancer Society)**

Isn't that a great visual? Cancer cells committing suicide!

Another interesting side effect of taking high doses of Prednisone is a remarkable surge in energy, something I didn't count on. That extra energy, though, did help me reach one of my chemotherapy goals. As I've said, I wanted to be physically stronger at the end of chemo than at the beginning. In fact, during one of my regular CT scans, the technician asked if I was a weight lifter. No! She was just seeing the effects of my doing pushups while I was taking the steroid Prednisone!

Part of my exercise plan was to do pushups every morning, 86 to be exact. The number 86 was very significant and empowering to me because shortly after I was diagnosed with cancer, my beloved grandfather died. He was—you guessed it—86 years old. My grandfather was a very strong man. I am his grandson, with his genes, so I knew I could be strong too. Doing 86 pushups each morning connected me to my grandpa, and his strength encouraged me to press on in the fight for my life. Having an anchor helped me press on when I didn't feel like doing anymore pushups.

So Prednisone can mean a surge of energy. Dr. Justice had told me about this stimulant effect and, based on his own experience, warned me to be careful: "I was taking Prednisone for a sinus infection," he warned me, "and found myself enthusiastically trading stocks in after-hours trading on the internet—and I had no business doing that. It can make you feel superhuman!"

About two months into my chemo routine, I myself experienced energy run amok. As I walked my boys to their morning classes at school, I started a conversation with son

Austin's fourth-grade teacher. It turns out she was getting married. Years ago, my wife Barbi used to have her own flower business, and she specialized in weddings. Putting two and two together, in my Prednisone "high," I thought how great it would be to offer Barbi's services—for free, mind you—as a wedding gift to Spencer's young teacher. Needless to say, I made one woman very happy and one woman very angry that day!

Be Prepared: Negative Side Effects

Unfortunately, not all the side effects of chemo are this fun or amusing. Some are downright nasty. But I have found that knowing is better than not knowing and being unpleasantly surprised.

That said, I still hesitate to talk about the negative side effects of chemo because I don't want to scare anyone away from embracing this life-saving treatment. But if you're fighting cancer, you'll be dealing with side effects, so we need to have a serious conversation about them.

If you're anything like me, you put off serious conversations as long as possible because they can be hard and painful. But I learned that I can do hard, I can do unpleasant, and I can even do painful. And you can, too, especially when your life is on the line. Cancer will reveal marvelous strengths you never knew you had.

My biggest fear going into chemo was **nausea**. I had read Lance Armstrong's book, and the poor guy seemed to be throwing up throughout half the book. Awful! As it turned out, I experienced virtually no nausea whatsoever. I was given a miracle drug named Kytril, which Dr. Justice was instrumental in getting approved for commercial use. I would take one Kytril the night following my chemo and two pills the day after. No nausea, praise God!

I did experience complete **hair loss**, eyebrows included. As it turned out, I was told that I have "the head" for being bald. Whether that was flattery or not, who cares? I lost my hair for six months. But it all came back, softer than before and a little thicker. When Barbi asked me how I felt about losing my hair, I remember saying, "Maybe by losing my hair, I'll be more approachable by people who are facing cancer themselves." As I've said, I had no room for negatives in my life, so I was always looking for ways to turn "bad" situations into good ones.

A year after my chemo, I was coaching my son Spencer's basketball team. The mother of one of Spencer's teammates had been diagnosed with cancer and remembered from my once-bald head that I had battled cancer the year before. I was able to share with her my story, refer doctors, pray for her, and encourage her. God used my bald head to open a door and give me a chance to encourage someone that I might not have had—and He has coordinated many such connections in the years since.

Mouth sores. Yuck. There is nothing good about mouth sores. They hurt, period. I have nothing good to say about them. No perky anecdote. No warm-and-fuzzy God story. The same is true for **anal sores**. Sorry to be gross, but you may get those too. I now know why Tucks Medicated Pads were invented. They are lifesavers! Mouth sores and anal sores—bad side effects that you may just have to deal with.

Stomach pain. The high doses of Prednisone I was taking caused stomach pain that was at times excruciating. In fact, it was a point of contention in my relationship with God. I remember being so angry at God for not protecting me from this particular side effect. One time when I was spending a night at my dad's house in Hermosa Beach, I had a particularly bad episode. The pain had not subsided for almost two days, and I went ballistic. Finding no one else I could blame, I let God have it with both barrels: "What possible f--ing reason could there possibly f--ing be for me to have this f--ing, f--ing son-of-a-bitch f--ing stomach pain!"

Not my best moment. By the grace of God, I wasn't smited on the spot, and a few days later my pain subsided, as did my anger toward God. I quickly apologized for my meltdown. Shortly thereafter God asked me during our prayer dialogue, "Robbie, why do you still uphold my name? Why do you call on me? I didn't take away your pain that day at your dad's house."

I took a long moment to really think about my response. Finally, I replied, "Because I know that you love me, Lord, and that's enough."

Faith becomes real faith when we don't allow circumstances to sway us from what we know to be true about God.

Bringing It to God

If you're upset with God, tell Him! It's better to be honest with Him than to try to hide your anger. Jonah told God he was so upset with Him that he'd rather die than do the work God set before him. (Read Jonah 4 for a great story.) As I've said before, God can take a few on the chin; He won't shrink from your venom. God didn't run away with His hands covering His ears when I was upset with Him. God hung in there with me when I was at my worst. He took my verbal abuse, and He didn't need to do that. He didn't need to hear Rob Raban spouting off at the mouth.

But by His unending grace, God loves Rob Raban. He *loves* me. And God loves you too. And God hung in there with me to teach me many valuable lessons, one being that I'm a lot stronger and tougher than I ever gave myself credit for. God didn't let me endure pain for pain's sake. He let me endure pain to make me tough and to help me realize that if I can go through this hardship, I can go through *any* hardship. If God needs to teach you this lesson, He may allow some pain in your life—for your benefit.

And let me remind you: not all side effects are negative. I've told you about a CT scan nurse who told me that my chest looked like that of a body builder (a Prednisone side effect). Another time I lost feeling in my fingers and toes because of the Vincristine, a side effect called **neuropathy**. Glasses would slip through my hands and break because I couldn't grip things tightly, but I played the best round of golf in my life at the Babe Zaharias course in Industry Hills because I could barely grip the golf club. My swing was light and free, and I shot an 83 (ten strokes better than my average). God allows cool, great, endearing, tender, amazing, and sometimes even humorous moments to come out of pain, even **bone pain**.

How many can raise their hands and say, "I know what bone pain feels like"? I was given a drug called Nupogen to help stimulate immunity-boosting white blood cells that fight infection. If your white blood cell count isn't high enough, you could be at risk of serious infection. In fact, chemo patients are not allowed to proceed with their treatments if their white cell count is not at a certain minimum level. Your pelvic/hip region is the largest concentration of bone in your body and therefore where most of the white blood cells are produced. The side effect of the massive white blood cell production prompted by the Nupogen shot is bone pain. Imagine the creaking you might expect to hear when a ninety-year-old man bends over to tie his shoe. That is the creaky nature of bone pain. As son Colby's T-ball coach, I taught hitting, throwing, and fielding both fly balls and grounders. Grounders, for heaven's sake! For three months I creaked like a geriatric gymnast every time I threw or bent to pick up a ball. In retrospect, it's funny!

Fatigue? Not so funny. Fatigue doesn't hurt, per se, but it does limit your energy level and therefore your activities. Fatigue gets more pronounced over time. Fatigue sucks because you just lie on the couch wanting to sleep, but you're so tired that sleep doesn't come. Now, I'm all for resting and napping, but fatigue is different. It's flat-out unpleasant because it doesn't let you do what you want to do, which is to either do something or nap. What fatigue does do, however, is give you time to think. Fatigue gives you time to consider the big issues of life without the pull of work, or play, or naptime. Fatigue gives you time to be with God, and that is a very positive side effect of chemo.

"Draw close to God and God will draw close to you."

James 4:8 NLT

The good news is that God is stronger than chemo's side effects, and despite how angry I was with Him because of the pain I experienced, God showed me that I was stronger than the side effects too. God taught me a lot about strength and courage and persistence and humor and grace. And He taught me that life isn't always about getting my way and that sometimes I need to humble myself, accept my circumstances, and trust in His plan.

"We rejoice in our sufferings, knowing that suffering produces endurance; and endurance produces character, and character produces hope."

Romans 5:3-4 ESV

I can see now what I couldn't see at the time: the Lord used cancer as an opportunity to teach me about life…. About having faith despite circumstances…About enjoying life and its quirky unpredictability… About letting go of my perfectionism and need for control… About trusting in God, trusting in others, having a positive attitude, and persevering in hope.

God was growing and strengthening my character.

And isn't that what a loving Father does?

Chapter 9
Family, Friends, and the Internet

ONE OF THE MANY BLESSINGS OF MY CANCER JOURNEY WAS the unanticipated response from people who knew us and even people who only knew *about* us. I was overwhelmed by the outpouring of support from family and friends. They responded as if an alarm had sounded, beckoning, "All hands on deck! Rob and his family are in need!" I always knew I had friends in the community, but to see their love in action was truly humbling and life affirming. I wouldn't have to carry this burden of cancer alone.

Almost immediately a meal chain was established to provide dinners for us. I would never have thought of that, but what a blessing! Our close friend Debbie Spear coordinated a meal schedule that she managed so we could concentrate on our doctor's appointments and deal with the emotional stress of life with cancer. What a thoughtful act of service and love! And how nice it was for Barbi and me to come home from late-afternoon appointments and find a home-cooked meal waiting for us. Even now, years later, I'm in tears recalling this simple but profound act of love.

Home-Cooked Love

A home-cooked meal says so much, doesn't it? The person doing the cooking took time out of a busy schedule to decide on the meal, make a shopping list, purchase the food using their time and their money, take it home, unpack the car, and cook a meal. Then, once the meal is prepared, these dear folks get back in the car and deliver the meal to our home, usually with a note to encourage my family and me. That's a lot of work!

A home-cooked meal is a tangible demonstration of love. Jesus says that the second greatest commandment is "Love your neighbor as yourself" (Mark 12:31). In James 1:22, the Bible tells us to "not merely listen to the word… [but] do what it says." A home-cooked meal is an investment of time and care by the preparer, which makes it a very special gift. A home-cooked meal nourishes both body and soul, filling you up with love and gratitude. My heartfelt thanks go out to the many dear friends for feeding the Raban family, including my sister, Marci, who flew in from out of town just to cook for me. Your generous acts of kindness and sacrifice made Christ's love very real to me!

Another tangible demonstration of love was help with carpooling. With three young boys who had school, sports, parties, play dates, and sleepovers, we needed plenty of carpooling help. Our friends Dana and Tim Wetzel stepped up and took our boys wherever they needed to go. Dana felt strongly that it would be easier on our children to have one familiar face—rather than several different people—pick them up and take them to and fro. Again, I never would have thought of this gift of service, but praise God for the Wetzels! Their thoughtfulness and sacrifice of time speak volumes of their character, generosity, and love. Hillary Clinton famously said, "It takes a village" to raise kids, and that is even truer for families struggling with the burden of cancer. We Rabans couldn't have done it without our village.

Unexpected Acts of Kindness and Hope

Cancer definitely gives people opportunities to show their love for you. Such times of desperation and hardship can truly bring out the best in humanity, sometimes in unexpected ways. Consider, for example, my co-workers at Industrial Valco, a wholesaler of pipe fittings and valves headquartered in Los Angeles. When I learned I had cancer and would be losing my hair during chemotherapy, our branch manager Vern Preston rallied several inside salespeople, warehousemen, and even my grandfather to all shave their heads for me. Coming to work one day and seeing close to a dozen of my co-workers sporting bald heads brought tears to my eyes and warmed my heart. What a *selfless* act of support!

"Carry each other's burdens, and in this way you will fulfill the law of Christ."

Galatians 6:2

And then there was the time I was out of Nexium, the drug I took for the stomach pain. A pharmacist risked his job and gave me a couple pills for free despite the fact that he couldn't find my prescription in his system. He could see I was in pain, and he responded from his heart. Such tender mercy from a total stranger!

One of the more elaborate acts of kindness came from my weekend basketball buddies…. Every Saturday morning at 7:30, a group of guys from our neighborhood would walk to the community court for a morning of pickup basketball. We usually had enough for a five-on-five game, although the lineups depended on who was out late the night before or away on a business trip. When I began my treatments, I had to stop playing basketball in order to conserve energy and avoid injury. But this didn't stop the guys—some of whom I barely knew because I only saw them once a week on the court—from sharing their love with me.

Somehow the guys managed to steal my left basketball shoe from my closet. (Barbi undoubtedly had a hand in this!) The guys nicknamed my shoe "Lefty" (of course), and for the next several months these guys would send anonymous letters in the mail with polaroid pictures of Lefty in some faraway city, pleading for help, desperately wanting to return to the closet and his beloved Righty.

Lefty was squired to the Great Wall of China, Hawaiian

beaches, and even the White House. His pleas for help would arrive intermittently in an envelope addressed in letters cut out from a magazine in different fonts and sizes, the kind that psychos use in the movies to anonymously torment and threaten their victims. Lefty was photographed with everyone from a US Congressman to NFL cheerleaders to airline pilots in the cockpit (not an easy photo to get in our post-9/11 world). I even have a picture of Lefty with comedian Carrot Top. Each photo was inscribed with Lefty's plea for help in getting him safely home.

How cool is that! These guys from around the neighborhood, some of whom I only saw at our Saturday basketball games, went to the trouble of lugging around an old basketball shoe and imposing upon people across the country to "please take a picture with my friend's dirty shoe so we can cheer him up while he battles cancer." I get choked up just thinking about it. I so looked forward to getting those envelopes in the mail.

As I said before, one blessing of cancer is that it gives people a chance to step away from themselves and do something for a person in need—and that is a beautiful thing to be part of. Thank you, Greg Thomas, Ted Hyman, and Pete McKinley, for being my jock buddies and for showing your love in a manner like no other. You put a smile on my face and gave me something to look forward to. Thank you, thank you!

Submitting to Kindness

Allowing others to give to me and accepting their gift when I knew I couldn't repay them was, however, a significant challenge as well as a huge blessing. We human beings can get so caught up in keeping our accounts square with one another. We don't want others to do more for us than we will be able to do for them in return. So, it's a big adjustment to truly submit to the kindness of others.

But when you think about it, life is never an even 50-50 split. It's usually 60-40 and sometimes even more lopsided. Anyone who's married knows this. At any given time, one person is rowing harder than the other. That's what love is; that's what love does. We need others to row harder when we're tired, hurting, or unable—and, in fact, others need that opportunity to serve in love.

> *"Let each of you look not only to his own interests, but also to the interests of others."*
>
> Philippians 2: 4 ESV

True giving doesn't ask for or expect a return. To experience this kind of giving firsthand—to know that people were giving to me out of the generosity of their heart without any ulterior motive, any expectation of repayment, or any scorekeeping—almost singlehandedly changed my view of humanity. It's sad to admit, but I used to think that most people were selfish and out for something for themselves. I also thought that if someone did something nice for me, that person expected some kind of repayment. Cancer changed my thinking: I began to open my heart to the goodwill of others and to trust not only God more, but people more as well.

Occasionally, however, we'll find weeds in this garden of love, and we need to manage those weeds. Some of your family and friends won't, for instance, know what to say to you or how best to help you, and their words may fall flat on your ears and, on occasion, perhaps even pierce your heart.

The more inquisitive friends and family members will want to know everything they can about your cancer, do some research, talk to their friends and medical acquaintances, and then pass along the knowledge they've gained—all to help support you. Still others will have no compunction at all about telling you exactly what you ought to do in order to best survive your cancer. (Moms typically fall into this category.)

Regardless of what camp your friends and relatives fall into, this one thing is certain: you will be receiving offers of help and advice, solicited or not, and you need to be prepared to respond to these well-wishers who do love you, however imperfectly.

TMI

Google "cancer," and over 750 million search results will appear. Google "alternative cures for cancer," and over 18 million search results will appear…18 million!

Vitamin C mega dosing (www.cancer.gov)and protease enzymes(www.cancerfightingstrategies.com) to attack cancer, vinegar baths and juicing to help detoxify the chemotherapy (ww.organiclifestylemagazine.com), B17 and apricots for raising your immune system (www.newswithviews.com), tannic acid for decloaking (ted.earthclinic.com), curcumin, selenium, resveratrol, green tea, blueberries, and a whole host of antioxidants to slow tumor growth (www.livestrong. com)—the list goes on and on.

You could spend endless hours researching all the alternative medicines and beneficial foods available for fighting cancer. And for some people, exploring alternative cures or additional treatments is an important part of their battle against cancer. If you're so inclined, then more power to you!

For me, however, I quickly realized that in the short time I had to fight my cancer before it won, I could not become an expert in my disease. It simply was not possible.

For starters, with undergraduate school, med school, residency, and then time developing a specialization, doctors spend thirteen years becoming an oncologist—and that's just to start a practice! The collective wisdom of western medicine based on the experience of thousands of doctors and hospitals around the globe; on thousands of drug trials; on research funded by billions of dollars and conducted for years and years by thousands of health care experts and shared in thousands of symposiums the world over—this knowledge has been compounding for decades. How could I even begin to master that body of knowledge? Again, my strategy was simply to get the best doctor I could find and then plug into the networks, programs, and treatments that he recommended and that represented the best of western medicine.

I focused all of my energy on trusting God, trusting the oncologist I felt God had led me to, and following the plan Dr. J outlined. Energy spent searching on the internet was energy taken away from my investing all of my heart, strength, and passion into my treatment program and my healing. I didn't want to be conflicted about possible approaches to cancer, and I didn't want to doubt the regimen my oncologist had determined was the best way to cure me. I felt God had given me an anchor in Dr. Justice and his expertise, and I wasn't about to dislodge that anchor.

Some might think that this approach limits options and requires putting too much faith in a doctor. Perhaps, but I didn't see it that way. I believe God was calling me to trust Him and trust His plan. So I submitted to the Lord, trusted in the plan He gave me through Dr. J, and stayed away from the internet.

> *"Trust in the Lord with all your heart*
> *lean not on your own understanding;*
> *in all your ways submit to him,*
> *and he will make your paths straight."*
>
> Proverbs 3:5-6

But just because I was submitting in faith to the Lord's plan didn't mean my well-meaning friends and family would. I soon began to receive emails from loved ones about the latest "cure" for cancer.

As I mentioned earlier, with over a 18 million search results for "alternative cures for cancer," the number of nontraditional cures is virtually endless, but I didn't have endless energy for responding to these email reports of possible cures. I needed a gatekeeper.

The Gatekeeper

I soon recognized that, although getting calls and emails from people concerned for my well-being was deeply gratifying and encouraging, responding to them all took energy. "Robbie, I read that blueberries are a strong antioxidant and that eating them is good for fighting cancer," my mom said. My dad was concerned about my cholesterol (we have heart disease in the family), and I was eating fast food. I've told you that I'd expressed this concern to Dr. Justice one time, and he had chuckled: "Rob, we've got bigger fish to fry at the moment than watching your cholesterol." Dr. J wanted me to eat anything that would keep the weight on.

It's important to recognize the feelings of powerlessness our loved ones—especially Mom and Dad—may feel for us. If your mom and dad are still with you, remember that you are their special someone. And if you're fortunate enough to have parents like mine, they have poured their life's hopes and dreams into your well-being.

I'm told the deepest anguish a human being can feel is to lose a son or daughter. So, it's very important to be sensitive to your parents. You will probably never know the tears they've shed, the sacrifices they've made, the sleep they've lost, nor the prayers they've said on your behalf. So be thankful for your parents and be sensitive to their doting. I will be forever grateful for the love and support of my mom and dad.

That said, it takes energy to respond to our loved ones, and it's these special relationships that make having a gatekeeper particularly important. That gatekeeper will help you do the all-important work of focusing your energy and strength where it needs to be focused: on yourself and your healing.

It takes energy to consider their advice and compare it to the program you're on. It takes energy to listen and express gratitude. Unfortunately, my energy was limited, and I needed help. Barbi became my gatekeeper. She gathered all the helpful advice, communicated it with me whenever I had the energy for it, and then managed the responses so that I could rest for the battle ahead. Her job was not easy!

Barbi politely screened telephone calls and emails, she managed my commitments, and she didn't schedule anything without checking with me first. Barbi looked out for me and, when needed, would talk at some length with people to ensure that they were on board with our plan and respected the course of action we had chosen. Close friends and relatives can feel helpless when someone they love has cancer, and they desperately want to help.

Listening with compassion—even when Barbi herself was facing uncertainty and fear about losing her husband—was one of the biggest blessings Barbi gave me. By God's grace, Barbi managed this demanding dual role of being strong for me and strong for others.

One way—among countless—that Barbi was strong for me was her protection when I was dealing with one of the biggest side effects of chemo: fatigue. Some days you just feel really, really tired. You have to be careful not to get too worn down, or your white cell counts will go down and you'll be at risk for serious infection. Barbi made sure that I had the peace and the space I needed after chemo so I could focus on rest and recovery. She managed the household, my appointments, prescription pickups, our boys' schedules, doctor's appointments, mealtimes, bath times, bedtimes, everything.

I wrote earlier about marriage being a 60/40 split with each spouse taking turns doing more of the heavy lifting. Barbi did 99% of the heavy lifting during my battle against cancer. She denied herself in order to be strong for me, strong for our boys, strong for our extended family, and strong for our community. Barbi became selfless in her service to me and to others without expecting anything in return.

"A wife of noble character who can find?

She is worth far more than rubies.

Her husband has full confidence in her
   and lacks nothing of value."

Proverbs 31:10-11

Permission to Care for Yourself

As destructive as cancer can be, an interesting benefit is that it affords you an opportunity to learn self-care, something that had always felt a lot to me like being selfish.

I was very self-conscious: I didn't want to be or even appear to be self-centered and selfish. Furthermore, by nature I'm a bit of a pleaser, and pleasers can't afford to be too selfish, or they won't be able to please anyone. When I was young, I always wanted to please my parents and friends, but things changed after my parents' divorce when I was in high school. For a while I totally rebelled against this "being selfless" notion and embraced a self-centered lifestyle of drinking and partying, of doing only those things that suited my interests.

Once when I was in college, for example, my father needed help with some chores around the house. His mobility was limited because of his stroke, so his request was totally understandable and right. But I rarely made the trip without a bunch of foot dragging and whining about not wanting to go and about missing out on time with my friends. After all, it just wasn't fun to help Dad around the house—and I wasn't much better when my mom asked me to do chores. I just didn't want to help. And, after going on a date, if I didn't care for the girl, I simply wouldn't call her again. I wouldn't explain or anything. I didn't want to face any uncomfortable feelings, so I just wouldn't talk to her again. That's selfish, that's self-centered, and that's what I was for too long a period of time.

Years later, as I began to mature (due in great part to getting married and to my growing faith in Christ), the pendulum swung the other way. Now I was looking out for my wife, my three boys, my business. Now I was totally looking out for others. My need to swing back to a self-centered mode—even for as valid a reason as life-threatening cancer—felt wrong and even shameful, and these feelings created an obstacle I had to deal with.

To be specific, I needed to give myself permission to take care of myself and not see it as selfishness. Self-care was critical: I needed to do what only I could do about my health, my needs, my rest, and my recovery without the attendant feeling of selfishness reminiscent of my adolescent version of self-care.

This time my focus on myself wasn't harmful to others; nor was it characterized by a bad attitude. But I definitely needed to sort this out. I needed to delineate the differences between self-care and selfishness; I could not entertain even the slightest notion that when I focused on battling cancer, I was reverting to an immaturity that caused others pain.

Why was this season of self-centeredness so important? Because—literally—my life depended on it. My being a martyr wouldn't have helped my family; acting the martyr won't help anyone's family. Furthermore, self-care doesn't mean being rude or inconsiderate. It does, however, mean verbalizing and standing up for your needs, establishing and maintaining your boundaries, and doing for yourself whatever you need to do to fight and win this battle. Letting the focus of this period of your life become all about you may be a challenge, especially if you're a people-pleaser, but it is imperative. You need to concentrate all your energy and effort on beating cancer. Cure is your highest priority!

Fighting cancer gave me an opportunity to fight for myself, and I became a stronger man in the process. I began to listen to what my body was telling me. When I was tired, I stopped what I was doing and rested or took a nap. When I was sad,

I cried. When I needed something, I asked for help. When I couldn't keep a commitment, I would say so. I gave myself permission to lovingly respond to myself and to whatever my body needed, and I tried not to guilt myself into doing more than I should.

This sounds so simple, doesn't it? Yet how often do we truly live like this? The apostle Paul helped clarify how we should live and why:

> *"Do you not know that your body is a temple of the Holy Spirit within you, whom you have from God? You are not your own, for you were bought with a price. So, glorify God in your body."*
>
> 1 Corinthians 6:19-20 ESV

Being so focused on your own self-care may feel selfish, but this is a very empowering way to live—and if you're fighting cancer, this vigilance about self-care may be key to a victory, to being there for your loved ones in the future.

As any flight attendant will tell you, you need to put your own oxygen mask on first before you can help anyone else!

Chapter 10
Signs and Miracles

DURING MY CANCER JOURNEY, GOD BLESSED ME WITH abundant evidence of His presence with me, with probably more signs and miracles than I could recount or than I even recognized.

In addition to the three I've chosen to write about below are the literally countless "ordinary" miracles that were occurring almost daily—miracles such as my changing belief about humanity; my witnessing the very best in people as unselfish and caring; having people make meals for us, drive our kids to their sports and activities, go on doctors' visits with me, call in favors from others on my behalf, shave their heads for me in support, give up meals and fast as they prayed for me, take a dirty basketball shoe and fly it halfway around the world to send me pictures and notes of hope and encouragement; having doctors' appointments go smoothly and be pain free, being blessed with a prayer dialogue with

God as rich as I've ever had, experiencing a connection and openness with others I'd never experienced before, being a bolder witness for Jesus than I'd ever been, and being totally convicted that God is REAL, ACTIVE, and LOVING because I experienced it.

Now these may not technically be miracles, but they impacted me as much or more than any miracle ever could. These were signs that God was watching out for me through the care and love of others. What rich blessings God poured out on me!

The Power of Prayer

I was nervous about my first chemotherapy, and I was really worried that I would vomit. Sorry to be gross, but I'd prefer to have a broken leg than suffer from nausea.

After I received my first chemo treatment, Barbi and I went to the home of our friends Charlie and Karen Koeller. (Yes, this was the Karen who went on our appointments with us.) She and Charlie had prepared a nice dinner for us—which I was unable to eat because nausea had begun to creep in. We gathered our plates and went into the family room.

While Barbi, Charlie, and Karen chatted and ate, I was encouraged to just lie down on the couch and rest. It was around 7:00 p.m., and I was tired from my day of chemo, so I put my plate down and closed my eyes. As I did, I began to relax and fell into a deep, comforting slumber, and with that slumber my symptoms of my nausea subsided.

I must have dozed off for only twenty minutes or so, but

it was a deep rest. I felt somewhat conscious of being there with the group, somewhat aware of my thoughts, yet in a satisfyingly restful state. When I woke up, I felt refreshed and rested—and hungry! I gratefully ate the chicken and salad Charlie and Karen had prepared. The rest of the evening passed uneventfully. Barbi and I said our goodbyes and returned home to sleep.

The next morning my mom called to ask if I had noticed anything unusual the night before. I remarked, "Funny you should mention it. Last night, around 7:00 p.m., we sat down to dinner with the Koellers, and I was unable to eat because I was feeling nauseous. Then I drifted off into this perfect, restful sleep, and when I woke up, my nausea and symptoms had gone away. Why do you ask?"

My mom excitedly explained, "My friend Stan asked his friends in Minnesota to pray for you, which they did. These friends like to lay hands on the person they are praying for. Since you were in California and they couldn't lay hands on you, one of them laid down on a table as a stand-in for you. Then the others laid hands on him and prayed for your healing."

"That was nice of Stan. You said they did this last night?" I asked.

"A little after 9:00 p.m., in Minnesota."

I suppose it could be a coincidence that my nausea left me at the same time seven brothers and sisters in Christ were praying over my proxy a few time zones away, but it takes a lot of faith to believe in that coincidence. That's the first miracle I wanted to share.

"Is anyone among you sick? Let them call the elders of the church to pray over them and anoint them with oil in the name of the Lord."

James 5:14

Another time I was lying down on my son Spencer's bed. The three boys and I said our nightly prayers together, and after telling them a story (part of our nightly ritual), I drifted off to sleep. While I was sleeping, I felt an unmistakable, deep depression at the foot of the bed, as if someone were sitting at the very end of it. Startled, I sat straight up, but no one was there. I looked at the boys' alarm clock, and it was 1:00 a.m.

I got up and started walking down the hall to our bedroom when, to my surprise, I bumped into Barbi in the hallway. "Did you just sit on the end of Spencer's bed? I felt something and woke up."

"No," she said. "But I fell asleep in the loft, and something just woke me up." We both noticed it was 1:00 a.m.

That was odd. For twenty-five years now, the nightly ritual has been for Barbi and me to watch some TV together and then go up to bed around 11:00 p.m. It was highly unusual for us to have fallen asleep in separate parts of the house, me in the boys' bedroom and Barbi in the loft. But asleep we fell, and we both awoke at 1:00 a.m.

The next day when we dropped Colby off at pre-K, his teacher, Mrs. Hypock, pulled Barbi and me aside. Intently, she asked if we had felt her praying for us last night. We looked at her quizzically, and she continued. "I woke up at 1:00 a.m. and couldn't go back to sleep, so I thought, 'Who can I pray for?' and thought of you."

Barbi and I looked at each other, "Yes!" we exclaimed. "Both of us were awakened at 1:00 a.m.," I said, "and it felt as if someone actually sat on my bed."

Mrs. Hypock smiled. "I visually hold people very tight in my arms when I pray for them."

You've got strong arms! I thought to myself.

Again, I suppose it could have been a coincidence that both Barbi and I were awakened by a physical presence at 1:00 a.m. in different rooms in the house at the exact time that Mrs. Hypock was praying for us, but—again—it sure takes a lot of faith to believe in that coincidence. That's why this is Miracle #2.

God's Emissary

Now Miracle #3.

One of the most threatening aspects of chemotherapy is the weakening of your immune system. Reduced immunity means greater difficulty fighting off infection. That's why chemotherapy patients can't be around people who are sick. Chemo patients can't afford to catch something that their body might be unable to fight off.

I made it successfully through my chemo treatments without any hospitalizations—until the tail end of my fourth month. I had been coaching and helping my sons' baseball teams and still maintaining a full workload. In fact, things had gone along quite smoothly for me with both family life and work—up to this point. Over one weekend at the end of that fourth month, while my oldest son Austin's Little League team was earning a spot in the Tournament of Champions playoffs, I was headed toward the hospital with a fever that wouldn't subside.

My temperature started rising slowly enough, but Dr. Justice, concerned about infection, had told us to call him anytime, day or night, if I ever got a fever. We called him when my fever quickly reached 100° F. He told us to immediately check in to the hospital. By the time we got checked into a room, my fever had moved up to 101°. I was quickly hooked up to an IV bag and given "broad spectrum antibiotics." As I laid down to rest, the fever seemed to subside for a bit, but I was still not feeling good.

Barbi was doing her best to cheer me up and comfort me, even lying down on the other hospital bed to keep me company. But in my feverish state, I couldn't relax, and I kept ruminating over stupid stuff. One of the nurses had commented that if Barbi stayed in the bed next to me, she would have to charge us. I didn't know if she was kidding or not, so I was troubled about paying for the bed. Our medical bills had already made finances tight, and I didn't need the stress. I began to get upset at Barbi—who was there to comfort me!

I was feverish, anxious, and feeling drained. I asked Barbi to pray for me—which she did. Later that night, after she went home to spend the night with the boys and get them ready for school the next day, my fever began to spike again. This time my 100° fever quickly rose to 101°…102°…103°… 103.5°… at which point the nurse called the doctor and asked what she should do. I was ordered to be packed with ice bags to reduce my temperature.

My fever was climbing past 104°, and my blood pressure had dropped to 85/44. My breathing was labored, and I really felt as if each breath could be my last. I remember being afraid—really afraid for the first time—that I might die. Whether I was close to dying or not, I *felt* like I was. No treatment or medication was working, my fever kept climbing, it was 3:00 a.m. in the morning, and I was alone and scared. All my strength had completely evaporated. I had absolutely nothing left. I remember telling God that I didn't even have the strength to pray and that He would have to handle this Himself. And God did, by sending an unlikely emissary.

Now my idea of a nurse is a kindly, compassionate, and caring female. Think *Florence Nightingale*. Now that is probably a sexist view, but I wouldn't be honest about this stage of my story if I said otherwise. That I had any thoughts at all at this point is amazing in and of itself. After I had felt like each breath would be my last, something suddenly changed.

A new nurse had arrived to take my blood, and he looked like no other nurse I'd seen before or have seen since. That's because the nurse God sent was a big, three-hundred-pound African American male whose name and face I can't remember. (You'd think I'd better remember all the details about such an imposing man!) He had an easy way about him, and he told me that he'd come to draw blood. I'd been having blood draws throughout the day so that doctors could try to determine why the antibiotics weren't bringing my fever down and hopefully prescribe ones that would. As I lay shivering on bags of ice, I really didn't want to get poked again in both arms. But with a 104°+ temperature, I had no energy to protest. I was utterly spent, but oddly my breathing became less labored, and I became less anxious.

God's emissary had huge, meaty hands. He gently grabbed my left arm to insert the needle and begin filling the syringe. His hands felt so warm against my shivering body that I was instantly comforted. It felt like the hands of God—strong, warm, and healing. I never even felt the needle slide into my vein as he drew blood. He mentioned that he had a girlfriend he'd been dating for the past seven years. I remember saying, "Seven years? Don't you think it's time to make an honest woman out of her?" He smiled and laughed. I smiled too as we shared a light moment. The nurse then walked over to the other side of the bed and drew blood from my right arm. Another warm clasp of his big, comforting hands, another pain-free poke of the needle, and then I drifted off into a peaceful sleep atop bags of ice and with my 104° temperature....

When I awoke the next morning, miraculously my fever was gone. A new nurse, the Florence Nightingale type, was taking my temperature. I asked about the male nurse I'd had the night before. She didn't recall seeing a male nurse during the shift change. "He was big, black, and three hundred pounds!" I exclaimed.

"I don't know of anyone working here who fits that description," she replied.

"You're kidding me?" I said. The nurse just smiled and shook her head no as she went about her business. Barbi came that to visit me, and I told her my remarkable story about the 300-pound male nurse. Astounded, Barbi went and asked the lead nurse on the floor about our 300-pound friend. The lead nurse looked directly at Barbi and said, "We have no one working at the hospital who fits that description."

Now, I know some people believe in angels, and as a Christian, I should probably believe in them as well. But truth be told, I haven't given angels much thought, and I admit I have trouble with the idea that they're walking about the earth giving us blessings. And it's quite possible that the nurse I spoke with simply had a shift that had never brought her into contact with my male nurse/angel—although one would think they would have seen each other. And I didn't know what to make of the lead nurse's pronouncement to Barbi. So I don't know for sure whether God sent one of His angels to care for me. But I *do* know that I drifted off into a perfect sleep and my fever left me after my nurse's beefy hands poked my arms with needles I never felt.

"Stretch out your hand to heal and perform signs and wonders through the name of your holy servant Jesus."

Acts 4:30

I hope the picture is starting to become clear. When you open up and pray to Jesus with "a *little* faith," you can expect miracles to happen. When I was all but spent, when I was unable to even breathe a prayer, God reached out His hand to let me know that He and He alone was strong enough to heal me. And God used His 300-pound black male nurse/angel whom no one at the hospital seemed to know.

I got out of the hospital the next day in time to see Austin get a hit in the Tournament of Champion finals. His team won, and the Rabans had much to celebrate. From where I had been a day and a half earlier, you can't imagine how good that celebration felt.

Chapter 11
Strategies to Beat Cancer

Cancer doesn't care who you are. Cancer doesn't care if you're young or old, handsome or pretty, in shape or out. Cancer doesn't care about your ethnicity, your gender, your religion, or your faith. Cancer doesn't care if you're rich and powerful or poor and destitute. Cancer doesn't care about your good works or lack thereof. Cancer is an equal opportunity invader.

When I was diagnosed with cancer, I didn't spend much time wondering how I got it. That wouldn't have helped me! And I didn't have the mental or emotional energy to go down that road anyway. Quite frankly, I was too terrified of my situation to invest energy in wondering how I had gotten there. And at the end of the day, who cares how you got cancer? It's an educated guess at best, and, yes, it's still a guess. For me, the only thing that mattered when it came to cancer was *how I was going to beat it.*

It's important to have a fighting spirit when you face cancer, and I pray you have this fighting spirit. It's also important to realize you're not alone. A world of resources and spiritual supporters are ready to come alongside you to fight the enemy with you—and to fight the enemy on your behalf! And while cancer itself is certainly not a blessing, it can and does bring blessings all around you. As I stated earlier, cancer can usher in a season of profound personal spiritual growth. I have no idea why God has allowed cancer in your life, but you can be sure of one thing, God will not abandon you when you call on Him.

"God is our refuge and strength, an ever-present help in trouble."

Psalm 46:1

Below is a series of strategies that were successful *for me*. They worked for *me*. They gave *me* comfort. They gave *me* hope. Everyone's experience with cancer is unique and personal. Strategies that resonate for one may not resonate with another. And while everyone is different, those of us battling cancer face the same enemy. So it is my hope that some of the specific strategies and tools that I used to fight and beat cancer will help you. My first step was to place my trust in God.

Strategy #1: Trust God and Give Your Cancer Over to Him

I did not want to die.

I did not want to leave my wife a widow.

I did not want my three young sons to grow up fatherless.

I did not want to fail….

I think the most important thing you can do when fighting cancer—or any life-threatening disease—is to first acknowledge that you need help and turn to God. Bring Him into the fight! Don't go this alone. Tap into the power that only the Creator of the universe can provide; ask Him for His power and strength. *Inviting God into the fight of your life is the single most important thing you can do to beat cancer.* Even if you haven't had a relationship with God in the past, humble yourself and ask for His help.

> *"Humble yourselves, therefore, under God's mighty hand, that he may lift you up in due time."*
>
> 1 Peter 5:6

After you give your cancer over to God, then openly share your fears with Him and with the significant people in your life. Do this as soon as you can—and don't hold anything back. The more emotion and honesty, the better.

If you have cancer, your time is precious, and you can't afford to waste time—and you'll be wasting time if you find yourself camping out on falsehoods like "I'm not afraid of cancer," "I can do this alone," " I don't need anyone's help" or, conversely, "Why bother trying to fight? I'm going to die anyway. God doesn't care about me" or other such nonsense. If you hear self-talk like this, know that it is Satan whispering. God is never the source of this kind of negative thinking. Be clear about who your enemy is.

I encourage you to be completely honest and let those tears fly. Those moments will be messy. That's OK. You can do messy! Think of it as finger painting. Remember finger painting when you were in preschool or kindergarten? It's messy business, but with the teacher's permission, any child can do it and the results are usually pretty good. So don't be afraid to get dirty with the emotions of cancer. Give yourself permission to let your feelings out and release your fears to God and to those significant people walking alongside you.

When I found out I had cancer, I cried and cried. I was so scared. And when I'm afraid, I—like everyone—seek security. Recognizing that cancer was bigger than what my shoulders alone could support, I realized how desperately I needed help. And not just medical help, but spiritual and emotional help as well.

My first call after Dr. Barnes informed me over the phone that I had cancer was to my wife, Barbi. Her love would be instrumental to my healing. My mom, dad, and stepfather Mike were there with me every step of the way, and their support was invaluable.

My second call was to my sister Marci and her powerful prayers strengthened me and helped me recognize that God is bigger than cancer. That awareness encouraged me for the road that lay before me: *God is bigger than cancer.* God would be with me throughout this battle. He had the power to defeat cancer, and He would equip me for the fight ahead.

> *"You have armed me with strength for the battle."*
>
> Psalm 18:39 NLT

"But what if I'm not sure about God?" you might still wonder. "What if God is just fiction, a distraction, a crutch, a fantasy?" If that's the case—and this may surprise you—be honest with God. Tell Him you're not sure if He cares or if He even exists! Tell Him that you don't believe He's even hearing you. And tell God—if this is what's on your heart—"I don't believe in You, God. Help me in my unbelief." And consider this: *Just because you don't believe in God doesn't mean God isn't real and powerful and willing to help you!*

Hear what God has to say:

> *"I am the LORD, and there is no other; apart from me there is no God.*
>
> *I will strengthen you, though you have not acknowledged me."*
>
> Isaiah 45:5

This verse of Scripture doesn't say that God will only strengthen never-doubting, ever-faithful churchgoing people. God is the God of grace. That means, among other things, that it's never too late to go to the Lord and ask Him for help. Humble yourself and invite God into your heart, your journey, your illness, so that He can save you—and save you not only spiritually from the consequences of sin, but also, if it is His will, save you physically from your enemy, the cancer. (I would encourage you to investigate Jesus' claims about His deity and the forgiveness of sins in the New Testament books of Matthew, Mark, Luke, and John. Also look back at chapter 7, "Have a *Little* Faith.")

Know this: God wants to have a relationship with you despite your unbelief. And God will accept you no matter what you're thinking or feeling. Even if you're a class A sinner who has thumbed your nose at Him most of your life, God still wants to have a relationship with you.

God's love and His power are available to everyone—and, yes, *everyone* includes you, whatever your story. So challenge your beliefs—or, perhaps better stated, your *un*beliefs—about God. Ask Him to reveal Himself to you. And rather than curse God for your circumstances, consider this option from the Bible:

> *"Give thanks in all circumstances;*
> *for this is God's will for you."*
>
> 1 Thessalonians 5:18

The Lord is not asking us to give thanks *for* all circumstances. That would be crazy! Thanking God *for* murder, rape, or cancer makes no sense at all. Instead, He is actually calling us to give thanks *in* all circumstances. We don't give thanks for cancer, but even when we have cancer, we can find reasons for being thankful.

We can, for instance, give God thanks that He is there to support us and that we need not fight this battle alone. We can give thanks for the truth that God wants to care for us, to bless us, and in, His Son Jesus, to save us from the eternal consequences of our sins. Again, we need not thank God *for* the circumstances, but *in* the circumstances, we can thank God for such blessings as the fact that He is there for us and with us.

So, I encourage you to be honest with God about your doubts and fears. Read what the Bible says, both the Old and the New Testament. Study the claims of Jesus and be open-minded as you do so. You just may find yourself drawn to God's promises and, as a result, choosing to hold onto them and to reject the world's cynicism. You may also find in yourself the courage to really trust God with your life and with your cancer.

Strategy #2: Have a *Little* Faith, Have a Plan, Follow the Plan

Don't complicate cancer. Yes, it's life-threatening, but that fact doesn't mean you can't beat it. God is bigger than cancer—infinitely bigger—so keep the situation simple in your mind: you have cancer, and you want to get rid of it. How are you going to beat cancer? **By TRUSTING GOD and the healing gifts He's given to people who can help you.**

You are not alone in this battle. A wealth of knowledge and

skill is available to you out there. Caring doctors and nurses have tools that can beat cancer and cure you! But you need to have a *little* faith.

> *"If you have faith as small as a mustard seed, you can say to this mountain, 'Move from here to there,' and it will move. Nothing will be impossible for you."*
>
> Jesus in Matthew 17:20

I was chided by Jesus to "Have a *little* faith." After I made the choice to trust Him, I then attended to the next two steps: *have a plan* and *follow the plan*.

> **Have a *little* faith.** "OK, Jesus, I can have a *little* faith that You can heal me. Not this big, perfect Abraham-type faith, but a *little* faith I can have. That's possible."
>
> **Have a plan.** Sure, God could miraculously heal me in an instant, but I felt led to get the best doctor I could, a doctor who was an expert in my disease.
>
> **Follow the plan.** I was going to trust the doctor God led me to and do exactly what the doctor told me to do. That's pretty simple, isn't it? Don't doubt, don't second-guess, don't whine and complain. Just follow the plan with confidence that God will heal you.

Have a *little* faith that God will heal you, find the best doctor you can to treat your disease, and follow the doctor's directions. **Have a *little* faith, have a plan, follow the plan.** With a doable plan and even a *little* belief, you will find the energy to follow that plan.

Strategy #3: Have a Reason to Live

OK, that three-step plan sounds simple enough, but what if the plan doesn't work? What if my doctor isn't an expert? What if I don't trust western medicine? What if it's my time to go and there's nothing I can do about it? What if I'm not strong enough to endure the treatments? What if, what if, what if… *What if I die?* Isn't that the real question in all of this?

Let me ask you a question: Have you decided to live?

I don't mean to be insulting, but this basic question is very important: Have you decided to live? Do you have a reason to live? For me, the thought of leaving my wife and three boys was so devastating and so terrifying that I couldn't possibly bear it. I was determined to survive no matter what I had to go through. The cost would be inconsequential. I would do anything, anywhere, anytime to beat this cancer. *Anything!* No pain would be greater than the pain of watching my young sons' faces if they had to say goodbye to their father. I shudder at the thought even now, years later. I would *not* leave my family alone. I would *not* leave my boys fatherless. *My family was my reason to live. My love for my family motivated to do whatever I'd need to do to survive.* What is your reason to live?

Strategy #4: Choose Faith over Reason

Use cancer to your advantage! With your life on the line, your priorities quickly become clear. And with your priorities clarified—you want to live!—hidden reserves of strength you didn't know you had will be revealed.

Consider the story of the ancient sea captain who upon landing on enemy shores would order his ships to be burned, thereby eliminating any hope his soldiers had of sailing away in retreat. This action signaled to his men that their only hope of survival was to win the battle ahead. Taking away any hope his men had of retreating to safety, the captain gave them a powerful motivation to fight to survive: they had to win the battle–or die. The men's *priorities were clarified*. The captain was not afraid to fight, and his men found out just how hard they could fight—just how strong they were—when their only option was to fight if they wanted to survive!

Let Jesus be your Captain! He's not afraid of a battle with cancer, and He's ready and waiting to help.

> *"He gives strength to the weary and increases the power of the weak."*
>
> Isaiah 40:29

Normally, our reaction to whatever we fear is to pretend it isn't there, so we don't confront it. But we need to confront our fear when we find ourselves face-to-face with a villain like cancer and our life is on the line. The bully named Cancer is like a team of circling sharks looking to eat you: they're looking for a fight, and they picked you! There is absolutely no escaping this confrontation!

You can't have a sane and rational conversation with the cancer sharks. You can't negotiate with them. Cancer sharks want one thing and one thing only: to take your life. Cancer doesn't "play nice," so you shouldn't either! YOU NEED TO FIGHT!

Yet some of us are afraid to fight. I know because *I* was afraid to fight! But God called me to fight and compelled me to fight by drawing me a picture. Actually, I drew the picture, but it was a picture the Lord had described to me. Here's a reprint of the picture I carried in my wallet:

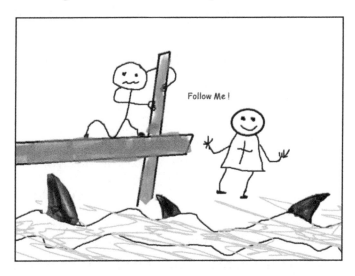

The stick figure hanging frantically as onto a piling atop a dock, as you might have figured, is me. Down below the sharks are circling in the water awaiting their next victim, and there's Jesus, jumping in with them saying , "Follow Me!"

The power of this image (outside of its obvious artistic quality- not!), demanded further thought. I didn't want to jump in the water because I saw the sharks down there! I also knew there were dead bodies down there that the sharks had eaten. Why would I want to jump in with them? And yet that was exactly what Jesus was calling me to do: jump into shark-infested water *with Him*.

So another question arose: "Who is this Jesus who is unafraid to jump into the shark-infested water?" The answer for me was that only someone stronger than the sharks and therefore unafraid of them would jump into the water where they were swimming! Translation: Jesus is stronger than the sharks! That belief gave me greater confidence about following Jesus and taking the plunge. I couldn't do this alone, but I could fight cancer with Jesus' strength and relying on the encouraging truth that He would be with me and He would fight with me.

> *"In this world you will have trouble.*
> *But take heart! I have overcome the world."*
>
> Jesus in John 16:33

But what about the odds of surviving the bully who is picking on you? If you're like me, you like to know in advance the odds of your succeeding, and that information can impact how much energy and effort you invest. If, for instance, your chance of success is high, you'll undoubtedly put more effort into the battle. But what if your chance of success is low?

How much effort will you exert, how much energy will you dig deep for, if your chance of success is well below 50%?

I concluded that the odds were irrelevant. Does it really matter if the odds of survival are 5% or 55% or 95%? You and I could survive—or you and I could die—whatever the odds, wherein lies my point: Will any attempt to have a rational discussion about the odds of your survival increase your chances of surviving?

Cancer gave me the opportunity to realize that *the odds are what you make them*. The battle against cancer is not about being rational or even logical. *The battle is about being faithful.* Regardless of what medical science has to say or what the latest stats are from corporate, are you willing to take the risk of trusting that the Creator of the universe can defy the odds and cure you?

> *"God's voice thunders in marvelous ways; he does great things beyond our understanding."*
>
> Job 37:5

Strategy #5: Think Positively!

I made the decision to live.

I made the decision that I would do anything I had to do in order to survive. Absolutely nothing was going to stop me. Yes, if it was my time to go, then it was my time to go, and I would have to submit to God's will. But I didn't believe that my dying was God's will at this point, so I didn't dwell on it. I knew that I wanted to live, and I chose to trust that God wanted to cure me. This was a positive decision I made.

After I made this decision, I focused my thoughts on the fight ahead. I chose positive thoughts of cure rather than any negative thoughts of loss. My mission was to focus on the thoughts that would heal me and suppress the thoughts that wouldn't. As I've said, giving your cancer over to God is a decisive first step toward defeating cancer.

If you fear you have the wrong doctor, pray about that concern—but don't waste valuable time worrying. Ask God to either confirm your choice or lead you to another doctor. Then, once you find your doctor, trust your decision and commit yourself totally to his or her program. Trust your doctor's expertise. I knew I couldn't become an expert in my cancer, so I chose to stay away from the internet and instead focus my energy on following my doctor's plan. I didn't want the internet to divert my focus away from the task at hand. I wouldn't learn in a matter of days and weeks as much as my oncologist had learned during the thirty-plus years of his study and practice of medicine.

Also, expect an assault from Satan. And I'm not talking about the cartoon Satan with horns and a pitchfork. I'm talking about the biblical Satan who whispers in your ear to doubt God and to go it on your own. Satan does not want you to rely on God. Satan doesn't want you to seek comfort in God or strength from God. Satan doesn't want you to be cured. Satan doesn't want you to have faith in God because he knows that God can cure you. Satan doesn't want you to experience God's power and of know His peace in your life. Satan doesn't want you to find yourself able to—by God's grace—stand up and be strong; Satan doesn't want you to fight cancer and win.

After all, what if everyone came to truly believe in God and His miraculous power? What would that mean for Satan and his evil works? Satan doesn't want an army of God-believers robbing him of his power by recognizing how truly weak he is. In fact, Satan wants you to believe that he doesn't even exist. Satan wants you to be rational, to pay attention to the odds, and to lead a dull, predictable life, pretty sure that God won't ever do anything grand for you. Satan wants to keep you mired in the shame-fueled belief that you don't deserve God's healing touch: *Why should I live when people better than me die? What makes me so special? People far better than me—people who were kinder, more generous, more patient, holier, more trusting, etc., etc.—have trusted God and He didn't save them! Why would God save me?* If you've had thoughts like these, you can be sure they are not coming from God! They are coming from your enemy, from the pit of hell itself.

When thoughts like these scream at you and demand your attention—when life isn't unfolding the way you want it to, when you're tired of all the bumps in your road, when you're frightened by circumstances and want to be comforted, when doubts and fears and anger rise up within you—how will you respond? In moments like these, it is time—more than ever—to choose to trust God. Invite Jesus to walk alongside you. He will help you face your fears.

At times during my battle, I lost strength, fear crept in, and I was filled with doubt. That's when God would speak to me through family, friends, doctors, and Barbi. What a blessing her faith was! When I faltered, her belief that I would be healed helped me believe, and I would once again be able to trust God. Also, know that God will answer your doubts through the thoughtful gestures of friends just as He did for me. As I've shared, it was great when my basketball buddies sent me pictures of Lefty in faraway places with ransom notes that made me laugh. For a few minutes, I could forget about cancer. God also encouraged me through my sons and their pure love for me: their love reinforced my commitment to fight.

Do whatever you need to do to think positively, stay positive, deny the negatives, and keep trusting God.

> *"Now faith is being sure of what we hope for and certain of what we do not see."*
>
> Hebrews 11:1

Strategy #6: Decide to Be Stronger at the End of Chemo Than at the Beginning

Commit to being stronger at the end of your chemo than you are at the beginning. Visualize this stronger you. Choose to believe that reaching that goal is absolutely possible. This strategy proved very powerful and effective for me—and one reason was that it countered my fundamental belief that everyone on chemo basically withers up and barely survives.

I know that many people have a negative association with chemotherapy. I understand why, but really, why? Chemotherapy is your best chance to defeat cancer and save your life. Make friends with chemo. Embrace it! Give your fear about chemo over to God. He's not afraid of cancer or chemo, and with all the anti-nausea drugs available, chemo is significantly more tolerable than it used to be.

As you turn your fears over to God, ask Him to help you be physically stronger at the end of your treatment than you are at the beginning. I wanted to be strong for my sons. I didn't want them to see me wither away and die, so I chose to make chemo a positive. I decided I would use the negative side effects of chemo to motivate myself to exercise hard and be stronger. So be strong, survivor! Win! Set some goals for yourself. Life doesn't stop with chemo—and who doesn't want to be in better shape?

So I encourage you to envision yourself being stronger after chemo. My goal of becoming physically stronger in the face of often debilitating chemo inspired me. Instead of trying to retreat from a negative, I had created something positive to strive for. I swam, I played golf, I played tennis, I coached, I walked, and I kept on exercising, but an interesting thing happened when I started doing pushups....

Strategy #7: Create Visual Anchors

In honor of my grandpa—who was 86 at the time of his passing—I started doing eighty-six pushups a day. And I created a powerful visual anchor for myself: I pictured his still-strong 86-year-old self, encouraging me as I did my pushups. After all that my grandpa done for me, I could at least do these pushups for him! By linking my exercise routine to someone meaningful, I found the strength to push on even when I didn't feel like doing so.

On a side note, as part of my chemo, I was given the CHOP regimen, the P standing for the steroid prednisone. This was a wink from the Lord because Steroids + Pushups = Big Pecs!! Honestly, my chest actually grew during my chemo. I mentioned the C/T scan technician who asked if I was a body builder because of the size of my pectoral muscles. I'm a pretty slender guy, and I can honestly say nobody had ever before confused me with a body builder. Needless to say, I was pretty stoked. Her comment inspired me to keep pressing on. Of course, chemo is tough, but you can use it and some of its unintended side effects to motivate you to be stronger than ever.

Another visual anchor I created helped me in the chemo ward. Whenever I was receiving my chemotherapy, especially the reddish, Dippity Doo-looking Adriamycin, I pictured my bones as solid pillars and cancer as sand loosely stuck on the pillars. I further visualized my bones being made of pure marble—hard, solid, slippery, and not allowing any cancer to remain attached to them. When the Adriamycin dripped into my IV, I visualized a river of chemo washing my bones sparkling clean, stripping off cancer as sand would be stripped off a marble column when hosed down with water. When I would urinate, I visualized dead cancer cells being eliminated from my body. The classic video game Pac-Man also gave me a powerful visual: I would imagine a Pac-Man named Chemo eating up cancer cells one after the other.

What visual anchors might help you? Try attaching each anchor to meaningful people or events in your life. Doing so will give you compelling and inspiring images that can energize you and enable you to more fully embrace chemo.

Strategy #8: Keep Working!

Working was one of the strategies Dr. J suggested to help me fight cancer. "You need to have a reason to get out of bed in the morning," he said.

I worked for my grandpa for fourteen years. He was my mentor and a great source of security for me personally. Strong physically, mentally, and financially, Grandpa ran Industrial Valco like a benevolent dictator, sometimes more dictator than benevolent! Case in point. Standing in the hallway one day, we had a minor disagreement over a work issue. When Grandpa grew tired of my protestations, he simply grabbed me by the belt and pulled me down that long hallway, past our corporate offices (yes, all could see), and finally into his office in the corner of the building. "Robbie," he said with his deep baritone, "if you don't like it, you know where the door is!" Message received loud and clear, Grandpa!

A day after my fortieth birthday, Grandpa died. It was a Sunday, and we had spoken that day about the crossword puzzle in the paper. I had given him a correct answer or two. He'd said, "Thanks, hon. See you tomorrow."

Well, I didn't see him at work on Monday. He passed

away that night, eight weeks after I was diagnosed and while I was undergoing chemotherapy. I was devastated. "Lord!" I cried. "How could You take away my grandfather at a time like this!" But I had no time to be devastated. Not only was I fighting for my life, but now I had to fight for our family business.

Although Grandpa was a great businessman, he wasn't a great estate planner, and we were facing a 55% tax hit on his estate. We were in danger of having to sell the business in order to pay the estate tax unless something drastic was done—and done fast.

In God's inimitable way, He chose this time of all times for me to take over the family business. I had huge shoes to fill and many new responsibilities. I definitely felt that God's timing was pretty lousy. Suddenly I had a lot of work to do!

Looking back, however, I can see that my being engaged with work to this degree helped me to not be overly focused on my chemo. In fact, many times chemo was just another appointment in a day full of appointments.

I also stayed on as coach for Colby's Little League T-ball team. Getting out and coaching a gaggle of five-year-olds was like playing at recess three times a week. Those kids gave me a chance to forget I had cancer and just play. What a blessing!

God knew the exact prescription for healing me. He kept me busy at work, and He surrounded me with the light and life of children. God kept my mind active at Valco as I attempted to solve some serious estate issues, and at the same time He gave me an opportunity to remember what it's like to have fun and play. God's prescription for healing may not be what you think it will be or what you want, but it will be what you need. All of this is to say, don't go into a dark hole if you've been diagnosed with cancer and other circumstances come crashing down as well. Trust God to use those struggles to make your life a more striking masterpiece that brings glory to Him!

Strategy #9: Invite the Kids into Your Healing

If you have kids, they will be looking to see how you handle this trial, to see how you rely on God, to see how strong God enables you to be as you deal with adversity. Be a model of courage. Give your kids an example of how to face life's trials. Key to that is telling the kids about the trial you are facing. Not everything, of course. Your five-year-old doesn't need to know you have a 25% chance of surviving cancer. Instead, answer your kids' questions and respond to their concerns in honest and age-appropriate ways.

Invite your kids into your healing process. Sometimes you'll be fatigued and can't do the chores you usually do. Give them jobs to do to help out around the house and thereby play a part in helping you fight cancer. Let them cheer for you when your hair falls out. My kids jumped up and down on our bed because hair loss meant the medicine is working!

Part of beating cancer is choosing courage. Nothing can prompt courage the way your kids' love for you can. Let your children's love motivate you to press on when you're tempted to let down or even check out. Be involved in their sports and schoolwork. Give them visual reminders that you're active and strong. Exercise! Go out and play! Swim and throw the ball, if only for a few minutes. Go ahead and really live life. Don't wait for your chemo to be over and then live the life you want. Give yourself permission to live that life—and to do so, use the energy that life-threatening cancer paradoxically gives you. You deserve to live life to the fullest right now—and your kids can be part of your doing exactly that.

Strategy #10: Have a Gatekeeper

Loved ones and concerned friends can feel helpless watching you go through cancer, and they may struggle to find ways to best help you. They will offer to do all sorts of things like take your children to school, sporting practices and games; to make and deliver meals; even go to doctor's appointments with you. The blessing of friends and family is huge, and you will need them in your corner for support as you fight cancer.

But the love and presence of family and friends can also be a burden at times, especially when they overwhelm you with advice on how best to treat your cancer. It's important to your healing not to let the good intentions of others keep you from staying focused on your plan. Having a gatekeeper—Barbi was mine—is a God-send.

Barbi fielded all the questions and concerns from my family and friends and left me in peace to focus on beating cancer. Barbi managed the meal plans, the kids' schedules, and the gracious friends who stepped up to help us out with these and other tasks. Barbi also offered her strong shoulder to cry on when friends and family members felt hopeless. Barbi shielded me from the emotional turmoil that others were going through so that I didn't have to contend with their feelings or carry the burden of their worry and fear. Having a gatekeeper gave me the emotional space to be fully invested in only my health and self-care. Literally, my wife helped save my life by clearing the space to let me fight for it.

In some cases your gatekeeper may be your parent(s). If this is the case, you'll need to have a loving conversation with them about *your* needs. This is your time for self-care, which may seem selfish. It isn't selfish; it's essential for survival. Once you've committed to your plan for treatment with the doctor you're partnering with, you can't waste energy worrying about what others think is best for you or trying to manage their helpful suggestions.

A gatekeeper can get everyone supporting your program by organizing their offers to help while shielding you from their well-intended demands. This will free you to get the emotional and physical rest essential to your battle. You're going to need every ounce of energy you have in order to fight your cancer. A gatekeeper will ensure that you have it.

Epilogue

IT IS A TERRIFYING TRUTH THAT CANCER CAN STRIKE ANYONE, but I pray you've found comfort and encouragement in the all-important truth that nothing is bigger than God.

I also hope you've seen that a battle against cancer can be a season of profound spiritual growth. Take advantage of it: Wholeheartedly embrace any treatment and any procedure you need. Choose to trust your doctors and nurses. Expect good results from western medicine and the amazing cancer-fighting, lifesaving technologies, procedures, and drugs the world's brightest minds have produced. Trust that God wants to heal you. Befriend Jesus, walk with Him through the unknowns that lie ahead, and trust Him to save you. In other words, make the decision to live.

And that means—as I've said before—embrace chemo. Visualize cancer cells being utterly destroyed by this amazing medicine you're being injected with. Get excited when you see nasty stuff being mixed into your saline drip because that's what's gonna kick cancer's ass. Picture the chemo drugs streaming through your body, washing over your bones and organs like rushing rapids on a wild mountain river—

cascading, turbulent, and powerful, washing away anything in its path. Embrace the half dozen times you'll urinate during a chemo session: the different hue of your stream means dead cancer cells are leaving your body.

The Blessing of Cancer

Barbi says, believes, and lives a life of "See it to be it"—and as I came to terms with my diagnosis, I decided I wanted to do exactly that: I wanted to see myself as the new face of cancer, energetically living life to the fullest even as I fought this life-threatening enemy. I wanted to see myself as strong physically, emotionally, and spiritually. I wanted to use the energy that the fear of cancer produced in me and make it work for me.

Yet at the same time cancer had quickly clarified for me a fundamental truth: I am in control of nothing—and that was a humbling realization. I recognized how desperate I was, and I truly reached out to God for help. Acknowledging my powerlessness enabled me to see more clearly God's tender mercies, His unending care for me and my family, and His abiding love, mercy, and supreme power. And when Jesus called me to jump into the shark-infested waters and "have a *little* faith," I was able to trust my life to my Savior more fully than I ever had before and experience His very real peace, love, and power.

> *"Have I not commanded you? Be strong and*
> *courageous. Do not be afraid; do not be*
> *discouraged, for the LORD your God will be with*
> *you wherever you go."*
>
> God in Joshua 1:9

During my battle against cancer, my view of humanity as well as of myself changed drastically. No longer did I believe that every person on the planet was entirely self-centered and concerned only about their own personal gain. How could I when I was experiencing caring, selfless, wonderful people at their best!

My wife Barbi is a God-send, and I will never completely know the extent of the sacrifices she made, and for which I am forever grateful, as she selflessly worked to give me both the space and the care I needed to fight my cancer.... Karen Koeller was an angel who joined Barbi and me at key doctor's appointments and chemotherapies, asking pertinent questions we failed to ask and writing down information we would have failed to remember.... People fasted for me as they prayed to the Lord for my healing.... My mom prayed unceasingly for me, cooked meals for us, and drove the kids to school and their various activities.... My dad had his church write me dozens of letters of encouragement, and he joined me at my chemo appointments when he himself was going through treatment for prostate cancer.... My sister Marci and her family prayed continually for me and my nephew Miles put together an encouraging scrapbook that gave me the powerful Jeremiah 32:27 scripture verse "I am the Lord, the

God of all Flesh. Is there anything too hard for me?... During this time my stepfather, Mike, stepped in for me and tutored my son Austin in math.... My friend Charlie Koeller was a continual source of spiritual encouragement and friendship (I love you, Charlie!)...

Countless friends cooked, drove, prayed, and helped out the Raban family any way they could. All of their tangible love and support gave Barbi and me an enormous amount of comfort. Tim and Dana Wetzel were especially helpful shepherding our kids around to school and practices.

My co-workers at Industrial Valco shaved their heads for me in a show of solidarity... My friend Dave Casey donated hours of his valuable time to help me process complicated business and estate tax issues when I didn't have the strength to navigate these alone.... I received cards and letters from people I'd never met who had heard about my condition and wanted to let me know they were praying for my healing.... I could go on and on and on about the kindness of others that was extended to my family and me.

My church family at St. Andrews Presbyterian in Newport Beach was an invaluable source of strength and comfort.... Senior pastor John Huffman offered his prayers and support.... My spiritual mentor Jim Birchfield, now the senior pastor at First Presbyterian Church in Houston, Texas, was a prayerful ally who—as a father of school-aged children—sympathized with my struggle and whose friendship strengthened me.

The Bible Study Groups that Barbi and I were a part of meant we had the support of brothers and sisters in Christ who were committed prayer warriors. In fact I would regularly feel them praying for me. My buddies Vince, Ted, Mike, Jack,

John, Allen and Dave would fast while they prayed for me! What sacrifices!

Clearly, I was not alone in my battle, and neither are you. But if you're feeling alone, contact a local church. Most churches can help connect you with caring, loving people to pray for your healing. A world of resources is out there ready to help you beat cancer!

As long as this list is, I will never know all the sacrifices people made or all the prayers that others have spoken on my behalf. So, in gratitude for those people who cared for and about me, I humbly offer this book. I pray that it will help and encourage others and, in so doing, honor those who gave so much to me, my family, and my healing. Because of the people whom God sent to journey with me, to fight *with* me, and to fight *for* me, I became a better person. Battling cancer helped expose and root out my limited, unfounded, and even wrong thinking about myself, other people, and my God. Battling cancer enlarged my worldview!

I trusted God with my cancer, and I saw Him move mountains—mountains of doubt, fear, anger, suspicion, self-pity, and selfishness. I experienced everyday miracles and huge, unexplained miracles. I experienced the love of the Father and of His Son, Jesus Christ. And because of God and the love of His Son Jesus, my faith has grown a thousand-fold, as has my love for people in general as well as for the precious individuals He has put in my life.

And I pray that you, too, dear reader, will experience these very same blessings—and more—as you fight an enemy that can be defeated!

God is ready to move mountains. Are you?

Bibliography

"Prednisone," Guide to Cancer Drugs at American Cancer Society website, last revised October 26, 2009, accessed July 28, 2014, http://www.cancer.org/treatment/treatmentsandsideeffects/guidetocancerdrugs/prednisone.

Savage, K. J., A. J. Ferreri, P. L. Zinzani, and S. A. Pileri, "Peripheral T-cell lymphoma—not otherwise specific" at PubMed.gov, published August 10, 2010, accessed July 28, 2014, www.ncbi.nlm.nih.gov/pubmed/20702104.

Szafranski, Michele, MS, RD, CO, LDN, "Weight Loss During Chemo," Expert Voices at the American Cancer Society website, published online January 24, 2012, accessed July 28, 2014, www.cancer.org/cancer/news/expertvoices.

Made in the USA
Monee, IL
28 June 2023